A Century of Radiology in Toronto

For my favorite radiologist,
Anne Marie Shorter, M.D.

A Century of Radiology in Toronto

Edward Shorter

Hannah Chair in the History of Medicine

Faculty of Medicine

University of Toronto

Wall & Emerson, Inc.

Toronto, Ontario • Dayton, Ohio

Requests for permission to make copies of any part of this work should be sent to: Wall & Emerson, Inc., Six O'Connor Drive, Toronto, Ontario, Canada M4K 2K1

Orders for this book may be directed to:

Wall & Emerson, Inc.	*or*	Wall & Emerson, Inc.
Six O'Connor Drive		8701 Slagle Rd.
Toronto, Ontario, Canada		Dayton, Ohio 45458
M4K 2K1		

Or by telephone or facsimile:

Telephone: (416) 467-8685 Fax: (416) 696-2460

E-mail: wall@maple.net

Canadian Cataloguing in Publication Data

Shorter, Edward
   A century of radiology in Toronto

Includes bibliographical references and index.
ISBN 0-921332-43-2

1. University of Toronto. Dept. of Medical Imaging – History.
2. Radiology, Medical – Ontario – Toronto – History.   I. Title.

R895.6.C3S56 1995   616.07'57'0711713541   C95-932149-7

Printed in Canada.

1 2 3 4 5 6   04 03 02 01 00 99 98 97 96 95

Table of Contents

List of Photographs

Abbreviations used in endnotes.

Hospitals:

HSC Hospital for Sick Children
MSH Mount Sinai Hospital
PMH Princess Margaret Hospital
SB Sunnybrook Hospital (after 1990 Sunnybrook Health Science Centre)
SMH St. Michael's Hospital
TGH Toronto General Hospital
TTH The Toronto Hospital (formed by the merger in 1990 of TGH and TWH)
TWH Toronto Western Hospital
WCH Women's College Hospital
WH Wellesley Hospital

Hospital institutions:

Board, trustees, etc. The respective boards of governors and the like.
MAB medical advisory board
MAC medical advisory committee

Other institutions:

CAR Canadian Association of Radiologists
OCI Ontario Cancer Institute
OCTRF Ontario Cancer Treatment Research Foundation
TRS Toronto Radiological Society

Journals:

AJR American Journal of Roentgenology
CMAJ Canadian Medical Association Journal
JAMA Journal of the American Medical Association
JCAR Journal of the Canadian Association of Radiology
NEJM New England Journal of Medicine

Preface

With the approach of the hundredth anniversary of Wilhelm Konrad Roentgen's discovery of the x-ray, it seemed appropriate to write a history of the Department of Radiology of one of North America's oldest and largest medical schools. Because academic radiology in Toronto has been conventionally parcelled out among a number of teaching hospitals, the task entailed writing not just the administrative history of the academic department—a relatively dry subject—but the story of the rise of radiology in the city's great hospitals as well. It is not an inglorious story, for Toronto took the lead in a number of areas of radiology and has to its credit a number of "firsts."

Yet I have not tried to write it as a history of firsts but as the tale of real men and women struggling with the challenges of the greatest technologic revolution ever to occur in medicine. For radiology changed the practice of medicine completely. Before 1895 medicine was the doctor with his little bag. With the rise of diagnostic imaging, medicine would depend ever more on fixed hospital facilities, requiring large staffs and substantial sums for their operation. Few fields within medicine were as caught up in technological change as radiology, where innovation occurred on an annual basis. Literally every year cash-strapped department chiefs and hospital boards would have to contemplate purchasing the fruits of scientific progress.

Managing this insensate pace of change required leadership. And herein lies the drama of the story. Leadership was needed to keep these hospital departments abreast of the state of the art, to ensure that the unique skills of the radiologist were not eroded by poaching from other medical disciplines, and to guarantee the provision of high-quality care. It is this story of leadership in the face of tremendous challenges that gives the history of radiology its particular fascination. Rather than chronicling the history of budgets, machinery and staff size, that is the story this book seeks to tell.

At the beginning, of course, radiology encompassed both diagnosis and therapy. In time, the two disciplines split apart. Radiotherapy became hived off into the Ontario Cancer Institute of the Princess Margaret Hospital while medical imaging continued as a separate field. In the present book the center of gravity is diagnostic radiology. Yet because the founder of radiology in Toronto—Gordon Richards—was primarily a radiotherapist I have decided to tell the history of radiation oncology in the city right up to the founding of Princess Margaret Hospital in 1958.

The records required for the history of radiology are widely dispersed. Although the university Department of Radiology retained little historical material, almost all of the eight hospitals that ultimately ended up in the university's teaching program have preserved the minutes of their boards of directors and their medical advisory committees. These various minutes together with the hospitals' annual reports provide the backbone of the story. In addition I consulted the archives of the Royal College of Physicians and Surgeons of Canada and of the Ontario College of Physicians and Surgeons, the Archives of Ontario, and the Archives of the University of Toronto, whose Department of Graduate Records provided information of great value. I was able to draw upon several private collections of papers as well. And the *Toronto Star* and *Globe and Mail* graciously made available the resources of their clipping files. Given this richness of material, it has been possible to put together quite a comprehensive history of the development of a medical discipline. But it is a history that features flesh-and-blood people acting to the best of their ability in often trying circumstances.

A number of people aided in this research. I am grateful to Erica Steffer and Mark Cave for their assistance with archival work. To Andrea Clark go my warmest thanks for administering the History of Medicine Program of the University of Toronto, in the context of which this book originated. And Susan Bélanger has my gratitude and admiration for her great skills as a researcher and editor. An earlier draft of the manuscript was read by Brian Holmes, Walter Kucharczyk, Edward Lansdown, Gordon Potts, and Anne Marie Shorter, and I am thankful to them for their meticulous comments and criticisms.

Edward Shorter
Toronto, 1995

Chapter One

Early Days

On New Year's Day, 1896, Wilhelm Konrad Roentgen mailed out reprints of his paper announcing the discovery of a new type of ray. Seldom has scientific news traveled so rapidly. Within weeks scientists and physicians everywhere were at work on the possibilities that x-rays held forth of visualizing the interior of the human body. Within days of learning of the discovery, young Harvey Cushing, then a clinical clerk at the Massachusetts General Hospital, wrote to his mother, "Everyone is much excited over the new photographic discovery. Professor Roentgen may have discovered something with his cathode rays which may revolutionize medical diagnosis. Imagine taking photographs of gall stones in situ—stone in the bladder—foreign bodies anywhere...."[1] In 1896 alone more than a thousand articles and 50 books were published on the subject of the new technique.[2] Just as Roentgen's discovery blew like a hurricane through medicine in general, it roared as well into the then very British world of medicine in Toronto.

Beginnings

Radiology first came to Toronto in January 1896, just weeks after Roentgen's announcement, in the form of a music-hall mountebank. A young man began to appear at the entrance of a theater on Yonge Street, Toronto's main street, with a small coil-type x-ray machine and a hand fluoroscope. For a quarter he would let the curious see "ghostly shadows of the bones of their hands on his screen." To convince bystanders of the virtues of his machine, he would first demonstrate the power of the rays on his own left hand. The fellow developed a severe x-ray burn and reported to the offices of Dr. Edmund E. King for treatment.

As King later said, "I'm afraid I was more excited about the way the burn had been suffered than the burn itself. I asked my patient to bring his mysterious outfit to the office, used it with a success that surprised me in the examination of one or two fracture cases, and later with a bigger and better machine used the x-ray constantly in my practice."[3]

King, then thirty-four, had graduated MD from the medical school of Toronto's Victoria College in 1885. He had an office on King Street East at the heart of town and staff appointments at the Toronto General Hospital and St. Michael's Hospital. King had behind him a long career in military medicine and was a prominent member of several Toronto medical societies.[4] He was, therefore, the perfectly situated person to introduce this revolutionary technology to the city's practitioners. On February 10 he gave "a very interesting talk" to members of the Toronto Camera Club on x-rays.[5] It is unknown if he reported any of his medical experiences but it is unlikely that he remained silent about them.

Meanwhile various other Torontonians were experimenting with x-rays. In these early days of February the story was of such magnitude that it was followed breathlessly on the front page of the city's various newspapers. By the first week of February, Dr. Charles Sheard, the city's medical officer of health and professor of physiology at the Trinity Medical School, had commissioned a photographer to undertake experiments "by which the interior of a human body can be photographed," as the headline writer put it.[6] Sheard was a graduate of Trinity Medical College in 1878, and had a practice on Jarvis Street.

The day after Sheard's work became public, a group of academics, including physics graduate student John C. McLennan (who later became professor of physics at the university), assembled an induction coil and a Crookes tube, the essential equipment for making x-ray images, and produced a radiograph of the bones of the human hand following an exposure of ten minutes.[7] Perhaps, forgetful of the sequence of events in these febrile weeks, McLennan later claimed that the photograph the group had taken days later (Feb. 11) of a Maltese cross placed inside a leather-covered

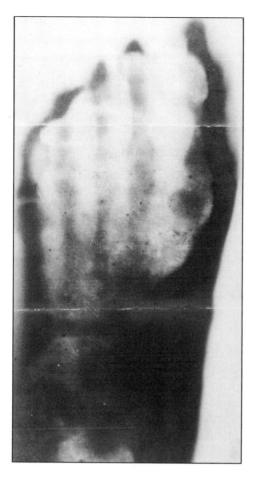

Figure 1.
The earliest surviving
Toronto radiograph,
taken in February 1896.
Obtained after a
30-minute exposure, it
shows the skeleton of
one of the university
professor's feet,
revealing a bunion.
*Canadian Museum of
Health and Medicine,
The Toronto Hospital,
General Division.*

box represented the first radiograph in Canada.[8] On February 12
another group attempted, unsuccessfully, to use x-rays in locating
a broken needle in a woman's foot.[9]

At the same time similar research was progressing in Montreal.[10] Indeed in the early months of 1896 frenetic interest in
Roentgen's discovery was being displayed in virtually every medical center and major city in western society.[11] In the international
world of "Roentgen's X-rays," boasted the medical press in March,
"Toronto and Montreal take no inferior positions."[12]

Two Hospitals

Clinicians in the Toronto hospitals were just as avid to acquire the new imaging device as those in the community. Ironically, the first Toronto hospital to possess an x-ray apparatus was the Grace Hospital, a homeopathic establishment, in February 1896.[13] Yet the big Toronto teaching hospitals, the Toronto General Hospital, then located on Gerrard Street East, and the Hospital for Sick Children, then on College Street, followed not far behind.

Of these two flagship Canadian hospitals, it was by a matter of months that the Hospital for Sick Children became first to acquire the x-rays. HSC was founded in 1875, and in the building on College Street that it acquired in 1892 there was space for 175 beds or cots.[14] Here the x-ray was an immediate hit. As the hospital's board noted in September 1896, "To show that the trustees are keenly alive to the progress of science, as applied to the healing art...our X-Ray equipment has just been imported from Europe, and this wonderful evolution of the scientific genius of the nineteenth century is added to the mechanical apparatus at hand. It will be sure to add to the marvellous cures already effected in this hospital."[15] The 1897 report stated that the apparatus "has been particularly useful during the past twelve months."[16]

Not only was the Hospital for Sick Children first with x-rays, it was first to have an x-ray department directed by a physician rather than a radiographer, or at least apparently directed, by Charles Rea Dickson. Dickson was born in 1858 in Kingston, Ontario, and went to medical school at Queen's University (MD 1880). He also studied for a year in New York where he collected another MD degree. Dickson then opted to return to Canada, preferring as he said "to live under the British flag."[17] In 1889 he came to Toronto to open an "electrotherapeutics" department at the Toronto General Hospital. (Electrotherapeutics, the peripheral application of mild jolts of electricity, was a therapeutic fad of the day and the forerunner of physiotherapy.) It was presumably in this capacity as electrotherapist that in 1890 the Hospital for Sick Children gave him a simultaneous appointment as "electrician."[18] He also had a private practice on Bloor Street. Dickson was not an inconsiderable figure on social and medical scene,

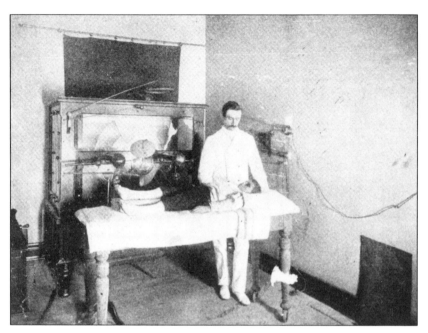

Figure 2. X-ray apparatus in use, Hospital for Sick Children, 1902. *Hospital for Sick Children Archives.*

being, for example, in 1896 one of the founders of the Canadian Red Cross. Yet it is unclear how much he actually had to do with radiology at HSC, for in those days physical therapy was often combined with radiology. Dickson may well have left the taking and interpreting of radiographs to the technologists, of whom a series passed through the hospital in those years. In any event it must have been under Dickson's aegis that a formal x-ray department was opened in 1901 at HSC.[19]

At both the Hospital for Sick Children and the Toronto General Hospital, the years before the First World War were more the period of radiography than of radiology. Toward 1900 at HSC, Mr. Stuart Jackes was noted to be "photographer and x-ray operator" (at a salary of $7.50 per week).[20] In 1904 G. A. Briggs followed as radiographer. In 1906 Dr. Samuel Cummings replaced the "electrician" Dickson in what was now formally entitled "The Roentgen Rays Department."[21] Cummings, who in 1888 had earned an MB from Toronto, was said to have worked with Roentgen, and had previously served as a radiologist to the Hamilton City Hospital.[22] It is unknown why he left HSC in 1907.

During the next decade the radiology department at the Hospital for Sick Children was run by radiographers, the last being Mr. W. A. Knox, until the appointment of Dr. Albert Rolph in 1919.

One of these radiographers played quite a significant role in the history of radiology in Toronto. At some point before 1910 Mr. Benjamin J. Fenner became the staff radiographer at the Hospital for Sick Children. Fenner was quite a catch, for he had trained with Roentgen himself at Würzburg in 1897.[23] He soon acquired an assistant, an orderly named Percy Ghent who worked in the hospital's pasteurization plant on Elizabeth Street and had become intrigued with Fenner's x-ray apparatus. Ghent started hanging around the radiology department and soon became a kind of apprentice to Fenner. In 1911 Fenner and Ghent were both lured away to the Toronto General Hospital and the Fenner era at Sick Kids came to an end. Yet the story is important because Ghent went on to become Toronto's leading radiographer until his retirement in 1946, and counts as the virtual founder of the discipline of radiography in Ontario.

Radiology caught on instantly at the Hospital for Sick Children because of its obvious utility in locating foreign bodies and fractures. In 1900 the hospital acquired a fluoroscope and in 1901 a new x-ray apparatus made (and donated by) the Edison Company. New pieces of equipment arrived constantly, for example, in 1907 a coil made by Wilhelm Scheidel & Company in Chicago, one of the earliest American manufacturers of x-ray equipment.[24] "The X-Ray apparatus forms to-day one of the most powerful therapeutic agents in the hands of the physician," intoned the trustees.[25] In 1902, 200 "sciagraphs," the contemporary term for radiographs, were made at HSC, in 1909, 890.[26] This was a more than four-fold increase in seven years.

When in 1910 Sir William Osler, the younger brother of HSC trustee and businessman Edmund Boyd Osler, came calling at the hospital, he pronounced himself "highly pleased with the progress made in this country with the x-rays."[27] Osler was then Regius Professor of Medicine at Oxford, arguably the most famous physician in the English-speaking world. This was not faint praise for the hospital's radiology department, the second oldest department of pediatric radiology in North America. (The oldest was established at Boston Children's Hospital in 1899[28].)

Meanwhile, radiology at the Toronto General Hospital followed Sick Kids a close second. Founded in 1819 and supported by the city, the province, the university and private donors, this thousand-bed hospital was among the oldest community hospitals in North America. After the University of Toronto Act of 1906, an advisory committee on relations between "The General" and the university was created.[29] It was determined that each professor in the Faculty of Medicine would simultaneously head a clinical service at the Toronto General Hospital. Therefore TGH would necessarily provide the main focus for the story of academic radiology in Toronto, as it did for almost all other teaching departments.

As the hospital's trustees contemplated the new radiology apparatus, they were a bit slow off the mark. In November 1896 they authorized the purchase of "apparatus for the Röntgen Rays for use in surgery, comprising coil, tubes, cells etc."[30] This marked the formal beginning, yet the equipment must have been inadequate for big tasks. To whom should surgeons at the General turn for help in locating bullets than—not the radiology service—but the professor of physics. In 1898, for example, a small-town family doctor wrote to Alexander Primrose, who had just become assistant professor of surgery, with a request for x-ray assistance in a gunshot-wound case. Primrose replied, "Dear Dr. Clutton, I shall be glad to do what I can for your patient if you bring him to Toronto. I have no doubt McLennan [soon to be the professor of physics] would be able to locate the bullet for us now that he has all the necessary apparatus." Primrose would be happy, he said, to extract the bullet after it had been located.[31] Physicists doing clinical x-ray work: Truly the discipline of radiology was not even yet on the horizon.

As at the Hospital for Sick Children, the early x-ray days at the General were dominated by radiography. After 1900, the trustees of TGH authorized the purchase of a great stream of x-ray equipment: a fluoroscope in 1906, for example, and an "X-ray stereoscope" in 1910,

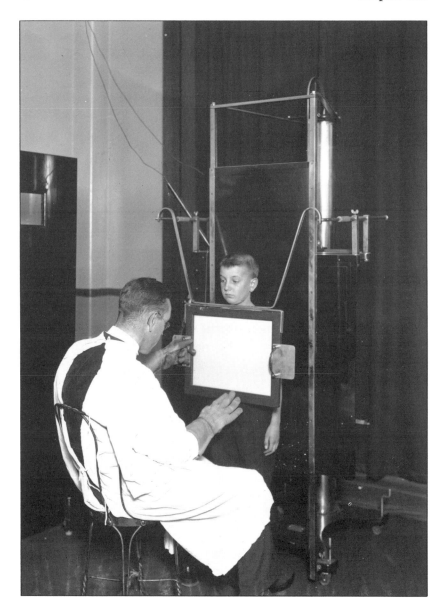

Figure 3. A fluoroscopic chest examination at HSC, 21 September 1917. Note the bare wires coming from the upper left. The hospital acquired its first fluoroscope in 1900. *Hospital for Sick Children Archives.*

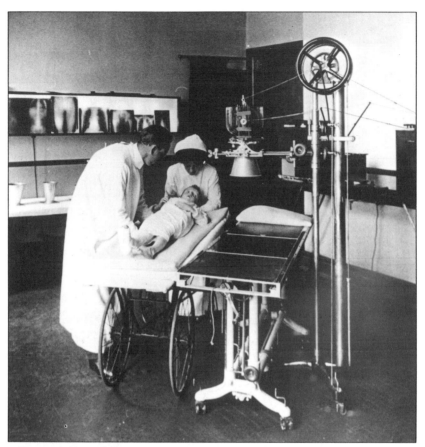

Figure 4. X-ray Department, Hospital for Sick Children, 1919. The radiographer is Mr. W. A. Knox. *Hospital for Sick Children Archives.*

all of it operated by radiographers, who apparently interpreted the results as well. In 1911 it looked as though TGH would finally acquire a radiologist of its own, appointing a recent medical graduate of U of T named James Harvey Todd (MB 1905). Yet later that year Todd's name was crossed out and that of radiographer Frank Fenner inserted.[32] It was this entry in July 1911 that first acknowledged the existence of a "Radiography Department."

In 1911 TGH had lured Fenner, and his assistant Ghent, away from the rival Hospital for Sick Children by agreeing to pay him half of the x-ray fees in addition to a salary of $500.[33] Driving back and forth in his old-model Ford with its elevated single seat at the rear, Fenner would simultaneously serve as radiographer for TGH, the St. Michael's Hospital, and the Wellesley Hospital.[34] He inter-preted the findings as well as making the films.[35]

At the Toronto General Hospital Fenner presided over quite a substantial operation in these years. After the move to the "New Hospital" in 1913, TGH would have a public wing on College Street and a private building around the corner on University Avenue. Each had its own radiology service. The public wing had all the hospital's physical therapy apparatus and an electrocardio-graph to boot. Indeed it was too much for a radiographer to manage. When on February 7, 1917, P. C. Larkin, vice-chairman of the board of trustees, proposed that Dr. Gordon Earle Richards "should join Mr. Fenner in operating the x-ray department," the era of radiology, as opposed to radiography, was about to begin.[36]

The Richards Era

The towering figure in the history of radiology in Toronto and in Canada is Gordon Earle Richards. It was Richards who founded the discipline of radiotherapy in the country as a whole, and who was the single most prominent national leader in radiology until his death in 1949. Here we give some account of his life and personality. The following chapter discusses his contributions to radiotherapy.

Richards was a quintessential kind of Upper Canadian figure, a combination of driving energy and British reserve. He spent a life devoted to work, a man who, as one biographer noted, "never learned how to play."[37] Born in 1885 in Lyn, Ontario, Richards was the son of a Presbyterian minister. His father, J. J. Richards, died of typhoid fever when Richards was four. With only a meager pension from the Presbyterian ministry, Richards' mother, Anna Paul Richards, "had a tough time to raise her family, two boys and an older one who died as an infant," as Richards' son Alan recalled many years later. "My father grew up without a father. I am sure he recognized at an early age that if he was going to get any kind of further education beyond public or high school he was going to have to arrange it for himself."[38]

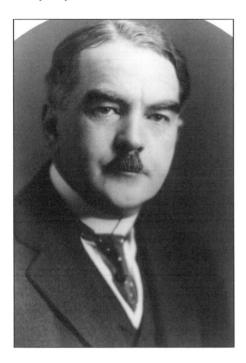

Figure 5.
Gordon Earle Richards
(1885-1949), the
"founding father" of
radiology and
radiotheraphy in
Canada.

Though born in Lyn, Richards grew up in Newboro, Ontario, in the home of a grandmother. As there was no high school in Newboro he commuted on a weekly basis to Athens. "He recognized that for university he was going to have to do it himself. So this made him a hard-driving, success-oriented guy," said Alan. "This was the way I pictured him all through his life. Success was paramount to him. Out to be the best there could possibly be."

His mother wanted him to be a minister, but Richards felt that his voice was too light. He decided to become a doctor, working his way through university and serving during holidays as a ship's purser. When he graduated in medicine from the University of Toronto in 1908, it was as the Gold Medalist of his class, the top-ranked student.

Radiology was not at that moment the number one subject on his mind. He went out to British Columbia to prospect for gold and serve as a mining-camp doctor. (He later sold his stake for $15,000, an unfortunately premature move it turned out as the stake became one of the largest gold mines in British Columbia.[39])

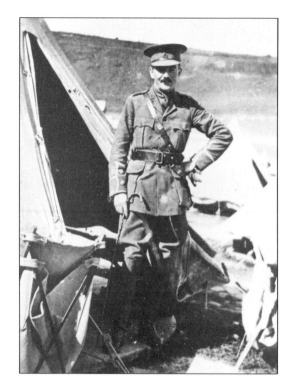

Figure 6.
Richards in the
Royal Army Medical
Corps at Aldershot,
England, 1915.
*Photograph taken
by Professor
Emeritus A. Murray
Drennan.*

In these mining-camp days he must have had some kind of experience with radiology, for in 1912 St. Paul's Hospital in Vancouver appointed him as radiologist. He was then joined in Vancouver by his University of Toronto classmate Charles Wesley Prowd (who also later became a distinguished national figure in radiology).[40] As World War I broke out, Richards and Prowd, both eager to go off to combat, tossed a coin. Richards won and Prowd agreed to stay on in Vancouver.[41]

Richards went off to war in 1914 at age twenty-nine with the Canadian forces. A captain, he was stationed with the No. 21 General Hospital of the Royal Army Medical Corps at various bases in Egypt. These years saw the beginnings of his scientific involvement in radiology. In 1916 he penned an interesting little note in the *British Medical Journal* on the radiologic localization of foreign bodies. Reflecting the pressures of combat surgery Richards commented, "One of the chief virtues of this method is speed, which is important when a large amount of work is at

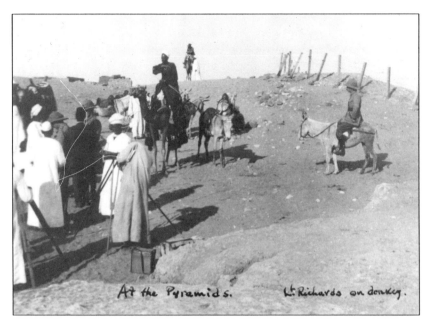

At the Pyramids.   Lt Richards on donkey.

Figure 7. Richards in Egypt, 1916. *Photograph by Professor Emeritus Drennan.* When shown this photo by Walter D. ("Bill") Rider, Clifford Ash commented..."Absolutely typical of Gordon Richards...you see Bill, he is astride traditional medicine, but unable to make it move, while his contemporaries are far too busy doing their thing...to help him." W.D. Rider, "The 1975 Gordon Richards Memorial Lecture," *JCAR,* 26 (1975), p. 175.

hand."[42] It is unknown why Richards was able to leave the Army during the war or why TGH singled him out as the medical man who should end the Fenner era.

"When he assumed command at the department," said Percy Ghent later, Ghent and Fenner were first to greet him. "Vividly, on that fateful day, his appearance is recalled. A straight, soldierly young man with fiery red hair appeared at the sole little desk then in use." The two radiographers decided that this individual looked too healthy to be a patient. "We asked him if there was anything we could do for him. He smiled, and his response came in the characteristic, semi-humorous manner that was to become so familiar. 'If things develop as I hope, you will probably be doing things for me for years to come.'"[43] Ghent became devoted to Richards and stood at the side of the casket at his chief's death in

1949. Fenner, by contrast, soon vanished from the hospital and the way lay clear for Richards to build a department.

What can be said of Richards' personality and character? He was a perfectionist with an iron-clad sense of duty, devoted to his patients though often brusque with them. One British visitor described Richards as "conceal[ing] his shyness under a certain abruptness of manner. With his short white moustache, bowler hat and trim, neat appearance, he had the air of a retired army officer."[44] Indeed, those who had worked with him recalled an almost authoritarian personality of the old-school, of which the Toronto Faculty of Medicine furnished other such splendid specimens as Duncan Graham, the professor of medicine. Radiotherapist Vera Peters used to refer to Richards "as a martinet in some ways, a man who set very high standards for himself and his staff. Some said he was very stern on the outside but soft and considerate underneath. He set a certain tone and manner of conducting the clinic."[45] Thus in the radiology department of the Toronto General Hospital the support staff did not address the physicians by their first names.

Yet the department was not exactly an ocean of tranquillity, for Richards could have a fierce temper. According to his biographer Margaret Shaw, "No one escaped entirely. Even those who had been on his staff for years and were among his most trusted associates sometimes found themselves the victims of his wrath." Remorseful at the outburst, Richards would then try to make it up to them, not by apologizing but by some small kindness. "His staff soon learned to accept these characteristic apologies. He was very impatient at times but his impatience was usually due to a failure in measuring up to his high standards. He lived up to his own standards and expected other people to do the same."[46]

Though some patients were intimidated by his brusqueness, those who were seriously ill cherished his display of concern. As Hattie B. of Buenos Aires, whom he had seen sometime during the 1930s, remembered him, "When I went to him for treatment I was very low spirited and had an almost incurable skin eruption, but with a year's treatment he cured me, not only physically but morally. He opened vistas in life for me when I was so totally

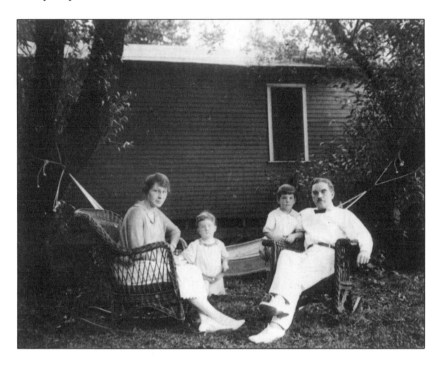

Figure 8. Gordon Richards and family.

discouraged, in such a fine fatherly manner that I have only the finest memories and thoughts of his noble character and kindly manner towards me."[47]

Is it little surprise that many of Richards' patients were attached to him? On Christmas Day he would go down to the cancer clinic in the Dunlap Building at TGH. According to the author of an unpublished biography, "One of the six- or eight-bed wards was cleared out for the occasion. A long table [was] set up and decorated, and all the Christmas goodies set out in lavish amounts." Richards would carve the turkey, making sure everyone got the part he or she liked best. "He was jolly and friendly and tried to make them feel happier and less homesick on the one day of the year when families particularly want to be together." Then Richards would push a "decorated hospital truck" with the turkey platter from room to room for the benefit of the bedridden. "Again he carved each patient's favourite part and stayed long enough for a few cheery and encouraging words." Then he would do the same thing at the Home for Incurables. After that it was on to the homes of "former patients whom he was afraid might not have too bright a day," the back of his car piled with "baskets and boxes of fruit, nuts, candy...books and magazines." Only then would he return to his own family dinner.[48]

In 1916 Richards married his childhood sweetheart Lila Isabel Singleton, the daughter of a businessman in Newboro. Of their three sons, Stewart was killed in the Second World War, mourned by the father until the end of his own life. After Stewart's death, Richards became increasingly remote and withdrawn from family life, experiencing little comradeship with his other sons and divorcing his wife in 1948. Shortly thereafter he married his head nurse, Claribel McCorquodale. Richards spent a brief interlude of happiness with her in a "dream home" he had built in the country near Weston, then died from leukemia the following year, in 1949.[49]

We return to 1917, where as the new head of the x-ray department of the Toronto General Hospital his first priority was to organize a proper radiology service. He immediately established an out-patient department, which in 1917 alone saw more than a thousand patients.[50] He organized the x-ray department into a gastrointestinal division and a "radiographic and therapeutic" division. He found it necessary to tutor the TGH staff in how to make referrals, and solicited "suggestions from the heads of other departments as to how the X-ray could be made most useful to them."[51]

In 1919 Richards initiated the department's first expansion by hiring William Howard Dickson as a specialist in the radiology of the gastrointestinal tract. Dickson was a McGill graduate of 1904 who, like Richards, had worked at mining camps in British Columbia. Unlike Richards, Dickson had sought systematic training in radiology in the States, studying gastrointestinal pathology with the well-known radiologist Lewis Gregory Cole of New York. (Dickson later helped pioneer the use of thorium dioxide.) Being said to possess an "almost oracular" diagnostic ability in the GI field,[52] Dickson soon made a name for himself in Toronto and was perhaps prevented only by his premature death in 1933 at age fifty-five of a

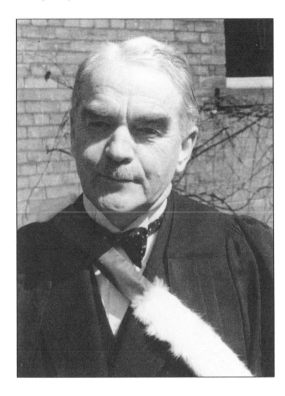

Figure 9.
Richards in later life.

heart attack from becoming an international figure. In the department, the division of labor would increasingly be that Dickson
handled the diagnostic side while Richards did the therapeutic.

The primitive state of equipment in those days meant that any
radiologist had to be a tinkerer to survive. One observer described
the early x-ray tubes as "globes of glass surrounded by zones of
profanity."[53] Richards had a long history of jury-rigging pieces of
diagnostic and therapeutic apparatus. In the early 1920s, for example, he and Dickson experimented with a special couch for con-
secutive gastric pictures. They designed a "complete serial gastric
unit" using roll film that incorporated thirty cassettes.[54] Over the
years Richards and his associates, particularly technician Thomas
B. ("Tommy") Hurst—an Englishman who had emigrated to Canada and in 1915 joined the engineering staff of the Toronto General
Hospital as an electrician—would devise many pieces of diagnostic and therapeutic equipment. Indeed, after 1919 Hurst became a
full-time technician in the radiology department.[55]

Turf struggles, an enduring theme in the history of any radiology department, began early at TGH as Richards endeavored to
defend his young discipline against encroachment. These are not
trivial matters for patient care, given that radiologists are generally
more experienced at interpreting images and that they do not
self-refer. In 1920, for example, the urologists demanded their own
x-ray equipment, and the medical advisory board of the hospital
thought fit to ask Richards' opinion. Absolutely not, he replied,
agreeing only to guarantee a room "at the disposal of the urological
Service daily from 9 a.m. to 1 p.m." The urologists backed off.[56]
Six months later Richards sent a signal to the entire hospital
staff—including almost certainly Duncan Graham with whom
Richards quarreled often over treatment—that he was in charge of
imaging and radiotherapy. He said that the chief of the x-ray
department would control the treatment of referred patients, and
"that in the event of opinion clashing with the physician or surgeon
in charge of the case," Richards would merely "discuss" it with the
head of the department in question.[57] These were major depart-
ment-building moves: Radiology would not be a cat's paw for
anyone.

Outside of the department, it was in these years that Richards
organized the first professional organization of radiologists in
Canada. In 1920 he convened eighteen colleagues in the board
room of TGH to constitute the Canadian Radiological Society. He
was its first secretary, and president in 1924. The organization
dissolved itself in 1927 to become the radiology section of the
Canadian Medical Association. (In January 1937 Richards
founded the Canadian Association of Radiologists, inviting radiologists from all over Canada to a meeting in Toronto.[58])

In sum by the mid-1920s, both within and without TGH,
Richards had established his presence. In 1924 the *Toronto Star*
referred to the x-ray unit of the Toronto General Hospital as being,
with the exception of the Mayo Clinic, "the largest and best
equipped department of its kind on the continent."[59] Gordon Earle
Richards, then thirty-nine, was starting to make his mark.

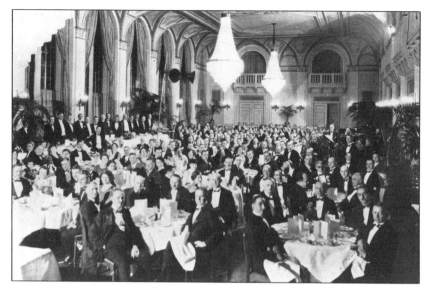

Figure 10. Banquet of the 15th annual Radiological Society of North America convention, Toronto, 5 December 1929. *Radiology*, vol. 14 (1930), p. 163.

The Two Hospitals Grow

The period between the arrival of the professional radiologists in the late teens and the rise of the subspecialties after the Second World War represents the founding years of Canadian radiology. At both the Hospital for Sick Children and the Toronto General Hospital these years saw great rises in the volume of service and an expanding support staff, yet almost no increase in the number of radiologists themselves.

No sooner would new office space become available than the multiplying number of machines would eat it up. At the General, radiology had gone into the basement of the College wing, or "Flavelle Wing," after the 1913 move. These dingy quarters soon proved too cramped and as early as 1923 Richards began planning for a separate X-ray building.[60] In 1925 the chairman of the board of trustees, C. S. Blackwell, began organizing a big expansion of the hospital as a whole. Radiology would go to the Dunlap Building, the pathology building on University Avenue that, thanks to a grant from the Dunlap family, had been renovated and named after the donors.[61] By November 1933 the radiology and urology departments were in their new quarters, urology on the third floor, therapeutic radiology with a fifty-bed unit on the second, and diagnostic radiology on the first. The little radiology department "rattled about like a few peas in a milk bottle" in the new space in the early 1930s (yet by the time they vacated the quarters in 1959 they would complain of "extreme overcrowding."[62]) With the move to the Dunlap Building, the radiology department left physical medicine behind.

At both HSC and TGH the distinctions among public patients who were indigent, public patients who could pay something, and private patients had been of great administrative and financial importance. Radiology treated the indigent patients from the city of Toronto free (about a third of the case load). To handle the overflow of private patients, in 1923 the trustees of the Toronto General Hospital established a private radiology office on Bloor Street, which then moved to the Medical Arts Building further west on Bloor Street in 1938. Because Richards had been instrumental in founding the building, radiology got choice space on the ground floor (where it remains to this day). This branch office at Medical Arts acted as "the private outpatient arm of the General," as Brian Holmes later put it, and the private patients' charts were interfiled with the rest.[63]

The enormous cost of imaging devices in the 1970s and after created the impression that radiology in the early days was somehow a low-budget operation. Not at all. In terms of overall hospital outlays, radiology equipment has always loomed high on the list and the trustees of the General were continually making special allocations for big purchases. It is to their credit that they almost never wavered, giving Richards what he wanted to keep the department state-of-the-art. For example, in September 1921 Richards requested $3000 for the purchase of "additional X-Ray equipment." The purchase was approved without discussion, despite the fact that, to the trustees' dismay, the radiology department was losing money and that this $3000 represented almost half of the total funds the hospital was receiving from its endowment in any given month that year.[64]

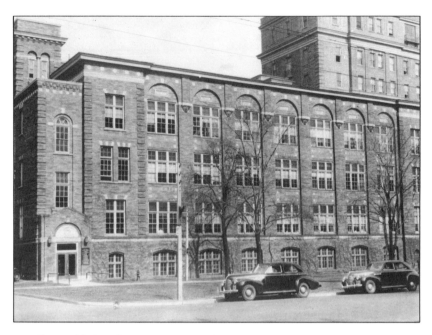

Figure 11. The Dunlap Building, Toronto General Hospital. By November 1933, the radiology and urology departments were quartered here, with therapeutic radiology occupying the second floor and diagnostic radiology the first.

At the time of the move to the Dunlap Building, the radiology department numbered eighteen support staff, including two technicians (evidently Ghent and Hurst) making $150 per month, four nurses making $76 per month, four ward aides, three cleaners, two clerks, one assistant photographer, and two orderlies (the latter making $45 per month).[65] Because Dickson had been ill since February 1932, the radiology department also included two young doctors whom Richards hired in May of that year: Arthur Singleton and Malcolm M. R. ("Mack") Hall. They completed the founding generation.

Hall was three years the younger, born the son of a physician in Brampton, Ontario in 1903. Graduating in medicine from Toronto in 1928, he had intended to become a surgeon but gave it up after an orthopedist tapped him on the shoulder in the operating room one day and said, "Son, you'll never be a surgeon."[66] So Hall went into radiology and, as a member of the triumvirate with Richards and Singleton, would look after the radiology office at the General.

Arthur Singleton, born in 1900 in Newboro and also the son of a physician, had a much more organic connection to the department of radiology at TGH. He was Richards' brother-in-law. Because Arthur Singleton's parents had died when he was about ten, he went to live in the household of his sister, Lila Isabel Singleton (who shortly thereafter would marry Richards). Although Lila Isabel had some money from her grandfather's estate, it did not suffice to send Arthur through university, and he, like Richards, was obliged to make his own way.[67] Singleton entered the University of Toronto medical school in 1917, left in the spring of 1918 to enlist as a private in a tank battalion, then resumed his medical studies after discharge. After receiving his MD degree in 1923, he trained in the United States, interning at St. Luke's Hospital in Minneapolis, then spending a year with Douglas Quick in radiology at Memorial Hospital in New York. It was therefore not favoritism (or favoritism alone) that prompted Richards to take on his brother-in-law. Singleton had a healthy American pedigree.

According to one account, Singleton commenced in some unspecified service at TGH in 1925, then joined Richards and Dickson in private practice in the late 1920s.[68] He must already have worked a lot with Richards, for when the Radiological Society of North America met in Toronto in December 1929, they conferred a special Certificate of Award on Richards and Singleton for unspecified "radiological studies."[69] Singleton's name first appears in hospital records relative to radiology at the time of his appointment to the TGH department in May 1932.[70]

Mack Hall was remembered as an affable man without distinction save among local organizations in Brampton. Singleton was remembered as a grand gentleman. A gentleman is not self-inflated. Edward Lansdown was a young resident when Singleton retired in 1962 at the age of sixty-two (when retirement as chief was mandatory). "I watched Professor Singleton taking down his name plate from his office door on the eve of the occasion. I said,

'It must be awfully hard to do that, sir.' He looked at me, smiled and said, 'No, it just takes a good screw driver!'"[71]

According to Brian Holmes, "Singleton was very charming with great social graces, urbane, a great sense of humor and a human guy. He was a man's man, very popular with peers."[72] Another colleague recalled him as "straight, honorable, old school. He chewed out a technician tremendously because she called him Arthur. Couldn't have that. British school type."[73] Alan Richards, a nephew whom Singleton treated almost as a son, recalled Singleton's "loud, genuine, enthusiastic laugh. He was well liked by peers and colleagues."[74] And indeed as Singleton and Richards began working together they seem to have got on well, brothers-in-law separated by an age gap of fifteen years.

As radiology established its utility in all branches of medicine, the work load of the department grew unremittingly. In May 1921 some 1300 patients were seen in the X-Ray department, by March 1937 over 2000 per month.[75] The trustees could authorize Richards to spend $25,000 for the purchase of x-ray equipment without batting an eye.[76] Radiology had clearly become a central feature of the hospital's life.

At the Hospital for Sick Children the radiography era ended in February 1919 when Albert Hill ("Bert") Rolph, at the time still at the Canadian army hospital at Basingstoke, England, was appointed radiologist. The medical advisory board of the hospital had recommended that "a medical man" be placed in charge of the x-ray department.[77] Unlike Richards and Singleton, Rolph was a man with an artistic side and wide cultural interests. Born in 1880 to a prominent Rosedale family, he had entered the U of T's general arts program in 1902, figuring prominently in the management of the student yearbook *Torontonensis* and in the student paper *Varsity*. He was said also to be "passionately fond of music" and to devote "all his spare time to his beloved violin."[78] Nonetheless, Rolph graduated in medicine in 1906, and after a year's internship at the Hospital for Sick Children went to London, England, where in 1909 he took the degrees MRCS and LRCP. He returned to Toronto, practicing family medicine until the outbreak of war. It was apparently during military service that Rolph, like many other Canadian radiologists, first cut his teeth on radiology. He was in the x-ray department of the Canadian base camp, at several English military hospitals, and at the Canadian Stationary Hospital in France.[79] At the behest of board member Sir Edmund Osler, Rolph was then hired as radiologist at HSC in 1919.[80]

Unlike the grimly dedicated Richards, Rolph remained something of a dilettante at radiologic work. In the judgment of his successor John Munn, Rolph was "a very nice fellow, a social person, he belonged to the Arts and Letters Club." Rolph was said to "like flowers, gladiolas. He loved kids. He'd rather go up to the wards and play with kids than do reports. He'd do his x-ray work but was always saying, 'Oh dear me.'"[81]

Yet Rolph had a powerful ally in the person of Leslie J. ("Les") Cartwright, an energetic and inventive Englishman who came to HSC as a radiographer at the same time. Cartwright had emigrated to Canada in 1910, studied radiography at the National Sanatorium's Gage Institute in Toronto under pioneer radiologist Frederick Peperdene, then during the war did x-ray work at the Central Military Convalescent Hospital in Toronto (where Eaton's College Street store would later stand). It was here that Cartwright got to know Rolph, and in 1919 he followed Rolph to the Hospital for Sick Children as radiographer (where he would remain until 1960).[82]

Cartwright has left us a picture of the radiology department at Sick Kids in these early days. It consisted of Rolph, Cartwright, and a secretary (who was not "under any considerations" allowed to take x-rays[83]). "The days of shockproof equipment had not yet dawned, so observers of fluoroscopy had to be warned not to get their knees too close to the wires under the table on pain of suffering a 60,000 volt shock. In spite of the warning…there were several incidents, one in particular in which one of our leading surgeons was knocked out for ten minutes." The radiology department also had responsibility for the hospital's photography. Continued Cartwright, "…In those days flash powder was used for photography and the heavy charge necessary for slow speed films created the effect of a small explosion which greatly upset Dr. Alan Brown [HSC's physician-in-chief] when he was lecturing in the adjacent lecture theatre!"[84]

If Richards imposed order on the medical staff of the General, it was the medical staff of Sick Kids that imposed order on Rolph. The medical advisory board was constantly admonishing him to do up a written report on each patient, "to be filed with the history," or to put the bulky glass plates on which radiographs were then made with the patients' charts (the impracticality of which suggestion he evidently resisted).[85] At one point the superintendent had to scold medical staff about removing patients' radiographs from the hospital.[86]

Midst all these growing pains Rolph decided in 1923 to go briefly on leave, and the person who counts technically as Canada's first female radiologist appeared on the scene: Lillias Waugh Cringan.[87] Born in 1890 the daughter of Alexander Cringan and Lillias Waugh, Cringan became MB at the University of Toronto in 1916, then moved immediately to Calgary where she served as house surgeon at the Calgary General Hospital. By 1918 she had left surgery and was functioning as pathologist and radiologist in Calgary. She returned to Toronto briefly to fill in for Rolph at HSC, at half his salary (yet with room and board in the hospital), then in 1924 moved to Ogdensburg, New York, to marry the Rev. William C. MacIntyre. Therewith Lillias Cringan vanishes from the Canadian scene. (She later became a psychiatrist, then chanced to die of a heart attack in 1967 while visiting Montreal.) Elizabeth Stewart of Women's College Hospital would go down in history as the country's first female radiologist, yet Stewart began radiology at Women's College Hospital only in 1919, Cringan beating her by a year as the first woman to do radiology in Canada.[88]

Under Rolph and Cartwright, the radiology department at HSC experienced great growth from the 1920s to the 1940s. The volume of work rose from 7600 radiographs in 1924 to 38,000 in 1946, the year Rolph retired. That latter year some 14,000 patients trooped through the department.[89] In 1934 another radiographer, Hugh Menagh, arrived alongside Cartwright. The department got its first intern in 1945, but aside from that there had been no increase in staff.

It was the efficiency born of ever newer equipment that made this increased volume manageable. But how was this equipment to be financed? Originally, the HSC board of trustees had the illusory notion that radiology would pay for itself. In 1919 the trustees declared themselves "confident...that a considerable revenue will be derived from plates and fluoroscopic readings for outside cases."[90] The trustees entertained the idea that prodding Rolph into doing research would be a money-maker. In September 1921 they convened him for an "informal talk...relative to the financial results at present being obtained by the X-Ray Department.

"There is no idea of faultfinding, or of making destructive criticisms, but the talk [has] the object of stimulating Dr. Rolph in the preparation of special papers to be read before the Faculty and doing special research work which will have the result of attracting work to the Hospital for Sick Children."[91] On another occasion the trustees turned down Rolph's request for a raise for Cartwright on the grounds that "sufficient effort was not being made by members of the X-Ray Department to attract pay patients."[92] Self-financing turned out, in other words, to be a disappointment.

Instead, in the interwar years at HSC, technological growth was financed heavily through private donations. It was a private grant that funded a better fluoroscope in 1929, for example.[93] But the great philanthropic Maecenas behind the growth of radiology at the Hospital for Sick Children was the Eaton family and the T. Eaton Company, one of Toronto's great department-store dynasties. This program of gift-giving began in 1919 as the employees of the Eaton firm decided to present Sir John Eaton with "a testimonial expressing their appreciation of his consideration for their welfare, and of the shortening of the hours in the store." Sir John indicated that he wished nothing from them personally but that the $20,000 they had collected be "devoted to the erection of an X-ray wing to the Hospital for Sick Children." As the presentation was made on June 24, 1919, at the Armouries, "where a great throng of the employees had gathered," Sir John said, "I hope the X-ray room will alleviate the suffering of the little ones. We all love children—God bless them. I hope that the all-day Saturday holiday will be enjoyed...."[94]

Perhaps the Eatons saw the gift to Sick Kids as a pendant to their endowment of a chair of medicine in 1919 at the Toronto General Hospital. In any event, it was an entire department they had funded with this initial grant: "The X-Ray Department donated by the employees of the T. Eaton Company is now complete," said the hospital in 1920.[95]

In 1929 the company gave again, followed again in 1940 by a very substantial grant from vice-president John D. Eaton for the refitting of much of the department's out-of-date equipment.[96] By 1950 the Eaton Company and Eaton family had donated $375,000 to the radiology department of the Hospital for Sick Children.[97] It is unknown why the Eatons had chosen to smile so warmly upon radiology at the children's hospital.

What rocketed radiology at HSC into public view in the 1930s, however, was not the kindness of the Eaton family but the Dionne quintuplets. Born in Callander, Ontario, in 1934 (and medically attended by HSC), the famous quints developed normally except for Marie, who had a hemangioma at birth and whose waddling gait suggested to the family physician, Dr. Allan Roy Dafoe, the possibility of a dislocated hip. Because HSC had acquired in 1934 an old army field x-ray to serve as a portable unit, Rolph and Cartwright were able to get views on the spot. In 1936 they loaded the unit into Rolph's car and trundled up to Callandar. "It was necessary to completely disassemble it to get it in the car," wrote Cartwright later, "and the transformer alone seemed to weigh about a quarter of a ton. We had dinner with Dr. Dafoe in a North Bay hotel and then started reassembling our monster. It was, of course, non-shockproof and was not really built for the fast exposures needed for these two-year-olds. The bathroom in the Quints' quarters had to be plugged up for light leaks and developing trays laid in the bathtub to see if our exposures were correct." The two

HSC staffers obtained, however, "some readable films" of their five celebrity patients.[98]

This era of growth in radiology at HSC ended on a bit of a chaotic note. The hospital had become aware of problems in the department. In 1941 the medical advisory board noted of the department's physical space, unchanged since 1919, "The over-crowding is appalling." "Out-patients have no waiting room except the hallway and private patients crowd into a room 7 feet by 11 feet." The main radiographic room had "no privacy except that afforded by some linen curtains. In-patients inevitably come into contact with out-patients [acquiring their infections]." Anesthesia for fractures had to be administered in the main x-ray room "with the result that the whole department soon reeks of ether, to the great annoyance of all waiting patients." The equipment was not shock-proof. Public patients had to share a single lavatory with private patients, a large concern then. Barium enema cases had to share that lavatory too. "The wooden floors of the department through which the outpatients are constantly passing are rarely clean in spite of constant attention from the orderly." Et cetera.[99] These problems were not necessarily Rolph's fault.

Yet the medical side of the service was tumultuous as well, as John Munn found when he reported for duty in 1945 as an assistant radiologist. "Rolph had lost control of the department," Munn later said. "Everybody else were reading their own x-rays. The doctors were taking their x-rays home. Pile after pile was located under their beds."[100] It was time for the beginning of a new era at HSC.

The early experiences of radiology at both hospitals call into question the notion that radiology was not instantly popular and that certain changes in the corporate culture of medicine were required before the device became incorporated in patient care.[101] To the contrary, in 1896 the culture of medicine in Toronto was primed and ready for an investigative means of such obvious utility. Toronto's hospital doctors leapt upon the new technology as soon as it became available. What arrived tardily, by contrast, was the realization that this special technology required specialist physicians to interpret its play of light and shadow. It took two decades for the specialty, as opposed to the technique, to be born.

Endnotes

[1] John F. Fulton, *Harvey Cushing: A Biography* (Springfield: Thomas, 1946), p. 104.

[2] A. E. Barclay, "The Old Order Changes," *British Journal of Radiology*, 22 (1949), pp. 300-308, detail p. 300.

[3] Quoted in Percy Ghent, "Highlights from Early Days of the X-Ray in Toronto," *Telegram*, May 25, 1949. See also obituary notice of King, *Telegram*, April 30, 1930.

[4] See King's obituary, *Toronto Academy of Medicine Bulletin*, June, 1930, pp. 14-15.

[5] "The New Photography," *Globe*, Feb. 11, 1896, p. 8.

[6] *Toronto Evening Star*, Feb. 5, 1896, p. 1. Sheard did not reveal the photographer's name to the press.

[7] *Daily Mail and Empire*, Feb. 7, 1896, p. 8. The others were Charles Henry Challoner Wright, a lecturer on architecture in the School of Practical Science (and founder of the department of architecture); Joseph Keele, a fellow in the school (who went on to work with the Geological Survey of Canada), and William Wallace Nichol, a fourth-year student in physics at the University of Toronto.

[8] Ghent, *Telegram*. On the events of Feb. 11 see the *Toronto Evening Star*, Feb. 12, 1896, p. 4. On the work of yet another University of Toronto group in early February, consisting of chemistry lecturer William Lash Miller (who would become the professor of chemistry) and C. A. Chant, a lecturer in physics, see the *Globe*, Feb. 12, 1896, p. 6.

[9] "The New Photography," *Globe*, Feb. 13, 1896, p. 10. The researchers were Dr. William H. Ellis, a physician and chemistry lecturer of the School of Practical Science, and Miller.

[10] See André J. Bruwer, ed., *Classic Descriptions in Diagnostic Roentgenology*, 2 vols. (Springfield: Thomas, 1964), vol. 1, p. 53, which, without giving exact dates, claims priority for Montreal in the production of Canada's first radiographs. On the debunking of the claim that the first clinical pictures anywhere appeared in Montreal, see Charles G. Roland, "Priority of Clinical X-Ray Reports: A Classic Dethroned?" *Canadian Journal of Surgery*, 5 (1962), pp. 247-251. It is likely that the introduction of radiology in the two cities was virtually simultaneous.

[11] On this rapid spread, see Stuart S. Blume, *Insight and Industry: On the Dynamics of Technological Change in Medicine* (Cambridge: MIT Press, 1992), pp. 21-22.

[12] Editorial "*In Re* Roëntgens' [sic] X Rays," *Canada Lancet*, 28 (Mar. 1896), pp. 251-252, quote p. 251.

[13] James T. H. Connor, "The Adoption and Effects of X-Rays in Ontario," *Ontario History*, 79 (1987), pp. 97-107, see p. 96.

[14] See *The History of the Hospital for Sick Children* (Toronto: HSC, 1918), p. 33.

[15] *Twenty-First Annual Report of the Hospital for Sick Children* (Toronto: HSC, 1896), p. 31. Hereafter cited as HSC, *Annual Report*.

[16] HSC, *Annual Report, 1897*, p. 5.

[17]D. C. Nesbit, manuscript biography, "Dickson, Charles Rea," submitted around 1960 to the Dictionary of Canadian Biography and kindly supplied to me by the editors of the *DCB*.

[18]HSC, *Annual Report, 1890,* p. 6. Here he is listed as "R. A. Dickson, electrician."

[19]Although the HSC *Annual Report of 1901* is silent on this subject, that of 1906 states, "Since the department was opened in 1901...." (p. 13).

[20]HSC, *Annual Report, 1901,* p. 5. On his salary see the minute books of the Board of Trustees of the Hospital for Sick Children, Apr. 23, 1900. These are preserved in the HSC Archives, and hereafter cited as HSC Trustees. Jackes resigned in December 1902.

[21]HSC, *Annual Report, 1906,* p. 3. From 1909 to 1912 Dickson belonged to the hospital's "consulting staff," but it is unknown what he consulted on.

[22]Personal communication from Dr. David J. Trew.

[23]"Marked Opening of New Science Era," *Globe and Mail,* Nov. 9, 1945, p. 15.

[24]See the HSC, *Annual Reports* for *1901, 1902, 1907.* On Scheidel see E. R. N. Grigg, *The Trail of the Invisible Light* (Springfield: Thomas, 1965), pp. 100-101.

[25]HSC, *Annual Report, 1907,* p. 9.

[26]HSC, *Annual Report, 1902,* p. 17; *1909,* p. 8.

[27]HSC, *Annual Report, 1910,* p. 9.

[28]On the department at Boston Children's Hospital see John Caffey, "The First Sixty Years of Pediatric Roentgenology in the United States—1896 to 1956," *AJR,* 76 (1956), pp. 437-454, detail p. 440.

[29]See W. G. Cosbie, *The Toronto General Hospital, 1819-1965: A Chronicle* (Toronto: Macmillan, 1975), pp. 141-146.

[30]Minutes of the Board of Trustees of the Toronto General Hospital, Nov. 2, 1896, p. 548, hereafter cited as TGH Trustees. These are preserved in the Archives of The Toronto Hospital, Toronto General Division.

[31]Primrose to Clutton, Apr. 9, 1898. University of Toronto Archives, Faculty of Medicine letter book, p. 158, accession number, A79-0023, Box 63.

[32]TGH Trustees, Apr. 5, July 5, 1911. See James Harvey Todd's biographical file in the University of Toronto Archives. He became a radiologist in the CAMC during World War I and died in 1918 following wounds he had received.

[33]TGH Trustees, Nov. 1, 1911. At this meeting it was officially noted that "Dr. Todd has been allowed to resign."

[34]Ghent, "Benjamin Joseph Fenner – A Toronto X-Ray Pioneer," *Telegram,* May 15, 1951, p. 6.

[35]Cosbie, *Toronto General Hospital,* p. 184.

[36]TGH Trustees, Feb. 7, 1917. The Trustees arranged that Richards and Fenner would receive two-thirds of the x-ray fees, from which they would pay the salaries of the department. The hospital would buy and own any new equipment.

[37]Margaret Mason Shaw, undated manuscript biography "Gordon Richards," ch. 1, p. 4. Ms. Shaw kindly gave me a copy of the biography, which will ultimately be deposited in the University of Toronto Archives. The manuscript is paginated by chapter.

[38]Alan Richards interview with the author, Apr. 27, 1994. The transcripts of all interviews conducted for the present study will be deposited in the University of Toronto Archives.

[39]Shaw, "Richards," ch. 1, p. 5.

[40]Arthur C. Singleton, "The Richards Lecture," *JCAR,* 4 (1953), pp. 29-31, 49-59, detail p. 30.

[41]Shaw, "Richards," ch. 1, pp. 5-6.

[42]Gordon E. Richards, "Localization of Foreign Bodies," *British Medical Journal,* 2 (July 1, 1916), p. 15.

[43]Percy Ghent, "Dr. Gordon E. Richards, A Tribute," *Focal Spot,* 6 (Jan., 1949), pp. 16-17, quote p. 16.

[44]David Smithers, "Hodgkin's Disease: A Review of Changes over 40 Years," *British Journal of Radiology,* 46 (1973), pp. 911-916, quote p. 912.

[45]Vera Peters communicated these opinions to the then junior radiotherapist Günes Ege. Ege interview of Nov. 15, 1994.

[46]Shaw, "Richards," ch. 4, p. 6.

[47]Quotation from letter of Hattie R. B——, Buenos Aires, undated, attached to manuscript of Shaw, "Richards."

[48]Shaw, "Richards," ch. 5, pp. 1-2.

[49]On personal aspects of Richards' life see Shaw, "Richards," ch. 11, p. 2.

[50]TGH Trustees, special meeting, Mar. 6, 1918, p. 3.

[51]TGH MAB, Jan. 3, 1921, p. 2.

[52]Percy Ghent, "Dr. William Howard Dickson," *University of Toronto Medical Journal,* 11 (1933), p. 46. See also Gordon E. Richards, obituary, *CMAJ,* 29 (1933), pp. 690-691.

[53]Barclay, *British Journal of Radiology,* 1949, p. 302, quoting Cuthbert Andrews.

[54]W. A. Jones, "Gordon Earle Richards—A Little About His Life and Times," *JCAR,* 6 (1955), pp. 1-7, see p. 5.

[55]See Arthur Singleton's obituary of T. B. Hurst, in *Focal Spot,* 17 (5) (1960), p. 284. Hurst retired in 1959.

[56]TGH MAB, meetings of May 10, May 17, and June 19, 1920.

[57]TGH MAB, Jan. 3, 1921.

[58]Singleton, *JCAR* (1953), pp. 29-30. A. Howard Pirie gives 1919 as the beginning of the CRS's existence as an independent association. "A. H. P.," "The Canadian Radiological Society," *CMAJ,* 17 (1927), p. 830. I am grateful to C. Stuart Houston for showing me a copy of his manuscript paper, "The Canadian Radiological Society."

[59]"X-ray Reveals Mysteries," *Toronto Daily Star,* Nov. 15, 1924, p. 2.

[60]TGH MAB, Apr. 30, 1923.

[61]See Cosbie, *Toronto General Hospital,* pp. 178-187.

[62]"Department of Radiology, Presentation to Interdepartmental Planning Co-ordination Committee, Toronto General Hospital," May 25, 1966, p. 24. Document in files of Department of Diagnostic Imaging, The Toronto Hospital, Toronto General Division.

[63]Interview with R. Brian Holmes, June 3, 1994.

[64]TGH Trustees, Sept. 21, 1921, pp. 183-184.

[65]TGH Trustees, Mar. 28, 1934, p. 836.

[66]Holmes interview.

[67]Alan Richards interview.

[68]Singleton obituary, *Radiology,* 92 (1969), p. 182.

[69]"Bestowal of Awards by the Society," *Radiology,* 14 (1930), p. 81.

[70]TGH Trustees, May 25, 1932, p. 725.

[71]Edward Lansdown interview, May 17, 1995.

[72]Holmes interview.

[73]George Wortzman interview, Dec. 14, 1994.

[74]Alan Richards interview.

[75]TGH Trustees, June 15, 1921, p. 148; Apr. 28, 1937, p. 1017.

[76]TGH Trustees, Dec. 4, 1940, p. 1196.

[77]HSC MAB, Feb. 29, 1919. A Dr. John S. Day had also applied for the post.

[78]Unsourced press clippings in his biographical file in the University of Toronto Archives.

[79]"Roll of Service," Rolph's biographical file, University of Toronto Archives, dated Dec. 24, 1919.

[80]HSC Trustees, Nov. 24, 1919.

[81]John Munn interview, Oct. 17, 1994.

[82]On Cartwright see "Profiles... Cartwright," in *Canadian Journal of Radiography, Radiotherapy, Nucleography*, 4 (1973), pp. 49-50.

[83]HSC MAB, Mar. 24, 1919. It is unknown whether this edict was issued because the secretary, Miss Haynes, had been doing radiography badly or because she wished to do it at all.

[84]Leslie J. Cartwright manuscript, "Reminiscences of 67 College Street," dated 1951, p. 1. HSC Archives.

[85]HSC MAB, Feb. 1, 1921; Feb. 24, 1922; HSC *Annual Report, 1922,* p. 38.

[86]HSC MAB, Mar. 14, 1934.

[87]HSC Trustees, June 20, 1923.

[88]Curiously, Cringan is not even mentioned in Rose Sheinin and Alan Bakes, *Women and Medicine in Toronto since 1883* (University of Toronto: Faculty of Medicine, 1987). Information about her comes from the Ontario Medical Register, from her personnel file at the University of Toronto Archives, and from an obituary in the *Toronto Star,* July 17, 1967. After her marriage she went by the name MacIntyre.

[89]See the HSC *Annual Reports* for *1924, 1946.*

[90]HSC, *Annual Report, 1919,* p. 6.

[91]HSC Trustees, Sept. 29, 1921, p. 172.

[92]HSC Trustees, May 13, 1924, no pagination.

[93]HSC, *Annual Report, 1929,* p. 62. From Mr. A. H. Green.

[94]Jesse Edgar Middleton and Fred Landon, *The Province of Ontario: A History,* vol. 5 (Toronto: Dominion, 1927), p. 662.

[95]HSC, *Annual Report, 1920,* p. 5.

[96]HSC Trustees, Feb. 5, 1929; Jan. 16 and Feb. 13, 1940.

[97]*Telegram,* Jan. 5, 1950, p. 1.

[98]Cartwright, "Reminiscences of 67 College Street," p. 3; Allan Roy Dafoe and William A. Dafoe, "The Physical Welfare of the Dionne Quintuplets," *CMAJ*, 37 (1937), pp. 415-423.

[99]HSC MAB, Feb. 10, 1941.

[100]Munn interview.

[101]See Joel D. Howell, "Machines and Medicine: Technology Transforms the American Hospital," in Diana E. Long and Janet Golden, eds., *The American General Hospital: Communities and Social Contexts* (Ithaca: Cornell U. P., 1989), esp. pp. 132-134.

Chapter Two

Radiotherapy

Although this book tells mainly the story of diagnostic radiology, the development of radiotherapy in Toronto enters in as well. Richards, the towering figure in the history of radiology in the city and in Canada, was primarily a radiotherapist. Here we follow the story until 1958, when the opening of Princess Margaret Hospital began a new era in cancer therapy the telling of which would take us too far afield.

Early Radiotherapy

The rise of therapeutic radiology in Toronto is basically the story of Richards' life. Yet it begins before Richards, and almost simultaneously as the history of diagnostic radiology commences.

On the heels of the discovery of Roentgen's x-rays there came in 1898 the no less astonishing news of the discovery of radium. "This was the signal for another pilgrimage across the ocean to the new shrine of knowledge," as one scholar put it, radium snatched up as avidly as the Roentgen rays.[1] Yet many fewer were the radium pilgrims because the substance was so costly. It demanded specialized centers and great financial resources. Even more than diagnostic radiology, radiation oncology would concentrate medical resources in a few large treatment centers. Radiotherapy meant a giant step indeed away from the doctor and his little black bag.[2]

The story in Toronto begins around 1910, when W. H. B. ("Henry") Aikens, a well-known Toronto physician with a practice on Bloor Street, began to use radium in the therapy of cancer and other conditions. He had been born in 1859 into a politically well-connected family, his father being the Secretary of State in

the government of Sir John A. Macdonald, Canada's first prime
minister. He studied medicine at Toronto, receiving his MB in
1881, then spent several postgraduate years in England and on the
continent. What drew Aikens to radium therapy is unknown. But
he was apparently close enough to wealthy patients as to have "a
large quantity of radium at his command" at his private Radium
Institute.[3] He was also on the consulting staff of the Toronto
General Hospital, though it appears that he did not actually do
radiotherapy in the hospital. As one of the earliest radium therapists
in North America—along with Howard Kelly of Baltimore and
Robert Abbe of New York—, Aikens used radium primarily for
skin cancers such as ulcerating basal cell carcinomas ("rodent
ulcers").[4] In 1916, he became the first president of the American
Radium Society.[5]

"Would you mind explaining the process of treatment?" a
journalist asked Aikens in 1914.

"Not at all," he said. He took from a velvet-lined case what
appeared to be a small seal, half an inch square. "There," said
Aikens, "is a radium plaque." It consisted one quarter of bromide
of radium, three-quarters of bromide of barium, "mixed with
varnish and put on a metal plate." These plaques came in various
sizes and shapes, depending on the area of the body to be treated.
The rays penetrated about three and a half inches, said Aikens.

Aikens also showed the journalist some radium drinking water
[sic], which she declined to try. "The use of radium in internal
medicine," he said is still very much in the experimental stage."[6]

At this point Aikens was the king-pin of radium therapy in
Toronto. What his response was to Gordon Richards' arrival at the
Toronto General Hospital three years later in 1917 is unknown.
But there is a soupçon of some tension between the two men. It
was upon Aikens' suggestion rather than Richards' that the board
of the Toronto General Hospital ultimately decided to acquire a
radium supply.[7]

Radiotherapy at TGH

The story of radium at the Toronto General Hospital began in 1917, when a member of the medical advisory board, the ophthalmologist D. J. Gibb Wishart, raised "the question of the total absence of radium in this hospital." Wishart said, "It [is] too bad that the principal hospital in Canada should be unable to give radium treatment." The board struck a subcommittee to consider the question.[8]

They pondered at length because of the staggering sums involved. Radium, a breakdown product of pitchblende, could be accumulated only after sifting great amounts of ore and cost at the time about $150,000 per gram.[9] Only late in 1920 did the hospital even get a quotation from a Pittsburgh firm that shipped radium.[10] Several months later, in January 1921 Richards and Dickson from the radiology department appeared before the medical advisory board to give them the bad news: 500 milligrams at a cost of $60,000 would be needed to produce emanation, or radon gas, to make radon "seeds" of glass or gold. (To keep this sum in perspective, recall that a staff radiologist made about $6000 a year.[11]) A hundred milligrams would be enough to treat one patient at a time. The board of trustees decided it did not wish to pursue the matter.[12]

Meanwhile pressure was building. The Faculty of Medicine was uneasy about the lack of radium at TGH. At the time that Richards was appointed lecturer, the curriculum committee noted that, "Radiology includes Radium-therapy.... At present there is no provision for such treatment or instruction in the Toronto General Hospital."[13] Staff from all over the hospital were demanding radium. In February 1921 the superintendent reported that he "has had many members of the staff approach him on the subject of the acquisition of radium for the Hospital." A minimum of 250 milligrams would be needed at a cost of around $30,000. Richards appeared before the trustees complaining that he was "compelled to refer far too many patients to cities in the United States because he has not the radium necessary to complete the treatment of the case." He demanded that another committee be struck: "If the Hospital is to maintain its foremost position among the hospitals on the continent it cannot afford to be without this very important mineral much longer."[14]

In May 1921 a private donor gave the hospital some money to buy radium and this, in connection with the sale of some of the hospital's land, created a fund of $20,000.[15] The radium arrived on September 9. It was such a big event that the hospital superintendent and Richards together made a public announcement.[16] The 150 milligrams of radium was not enough for emanation but sufficed to make the trustees exult by the end of the year that, owing to the soaring demand for x-rays and for radium, the radiology department was in the black.[17] The radiologists at TGH kept their $25,000 worth of radium in a small safe.[18] This was not just the idle pursuit of technology: In 1922 the first patient with cancer of the cervix was cured, living for sixteen more years.[19]

Meanwhile an entirely different mode of radiotherapy was establishing itself at TGH: high-voltage radiation, which involved passing 200 kilovolts and more through standard x-ray tubes. Although the hospital acquired a 120,000 kV machine in 1919, not until 1921 had Richards become sufficiently convinced of the advantage of this approach to press forward with high-voltage therapy. In that year he brought in a 200 kV device. In 1922 he got a second machine with a capacity of 300 kV, although it was never run at more than 250 kV.[20] One machine after another: the invoices came like hammer blows to the trustees, who by 1927 were starting to realize that radiology could be a very expensive proposition.[21]

Yet it was starting to pay off. In 1921 Richards became first in the world to treat pancreatic cancer successfully with radiation therapy. His first case was a fifty-two-year-old male whose carcinoma in the head of the pancreas had been diagnosed with the aid of a bismuth meal. The diagnosis was confirmed at operation in December 1920 yet no surgical removal of the tumor attempted. "The patient was then referred for deep therapy partly as a placebo, partly to relieve pain which was severe, and partly to test the possibilities of higher voltage treatment." That same month they commenced a series of treatments, another in January 1921, two months later still a third. The patient improved steadily throughout. At the present time, reported Richards in September 1921, the patient has returned to his normal weight, "and has carried on his regular business actively all summer. Roentgen ray examination shows no evidence of any mass, and he appears to be free from active disease."[22]

In 1926, re-analyzing the results of 37 patients with breast cancer whom he had treated post-operatively with x-ray and radium therapy over a period of four years, Richards concluded that radiotherapy had reduced relapses by about a quarter. "Any measure which...can be shown to improve the results of the treatment of breast carcinoma by 25 percent should be a welcome adjunct to the surgeon and the medical profession at large," he said.[23]

As a result of these successes, physicians in Toronto and elsewhere in the province were flooding the TGH radiology department with referrals, particularly for radium therapy. The number of cancer patients treated with radium at TGH rose from 494 in 1922 to 1321 in 1931, those with high-voltage x-ray from 553 to 897.[24] The hospital steadily bought new quantities of radium, only to see demand outstrip supply. 1926: "The X-Ray Department finds it increasingly difficult to meet the growing demands of the profession and the general public. The additional quantity of radium, viz., seventy milligrams, received on November 15th, is already in constant use...."[25]

This state of affairs clearly could not continue. The hospital was being inundated by cancer patients. In March 1930 Richards asked the medical advisory board to recommend that the hospital establish a Radium Institute to be situated in the Dunlap Building, the renovation of which was just at that moment being planned.[26] Seven months later fate took a hand: The premier of the province announced that he intended to establish a province-wide cancer service with clinics in a number of cities, including Toronto. The provincial government would pick up the cost of cancer therapy. The TGH put its own plans for a Radium Institute on hold.[27]

The Ontario Institute of Radiotherapy

In the late 1920s pressure was building across the province to increase the supply of radium and accessibility to radium therapy.[28] The rate of cancer in Ontario had risen from 70 deaths per 100,000 population in 1914 to 104 in 1929. In 1929 Herbert Bruce, the professor of surgery, called attention to "a matter of very serious importance, namely the lack of adequate radium supplies in this country." Although as a surgeon his first thought was not necessarily radium, he nonetheless felt that the half gram available in Toronto fell far short of the desirable minimum of two grams— and the province required nine.[29]

In June 1931 the Ontario government established a royal commission to report on the radium problem. Although it convoked a number of witnesses, the star was clearly Richards. He recommended the establishment of a cancer clinic in a general hospital, citing the clinic of the Philadelphia General Hospital as a model. Manifesting the Toronto-centrism that harvested him much ill-will among colleagues elsewhere in the province, Richards opposed the proliferation of cancer clinics in smaller towns.[30] When the commission reported in 1932, it followed pretty well the script that Richards had laid out: There should be cancer clinics in Ontario's three cities with universities (London, Kingston, and Toronto); they should be associated with large general hospitals.[31]

Over the months ahead, the province reached the following deal with Toronto General Hospital: the government would provide $280,000 worth of radium and as much emanation as necessary (manufactured in a plant in the Department of Physics of the University of Toronto). The cancer clinic in Kingston opened first in 1932. In November 1933, as the renovations to the Dunlap Building (which the province paid for) were complete, the radiology department of Toronto General Hospital moved into the first two floors. The diagnostic service was on the first floor, the fifty-bed radiotherapy service on the second. It was to be known officially as the Ontario Institute of Radiotherapy. The service was formally opened in March 1934.[32]

Richards wished rapidly to upgrade the therapeutic capacity of the service. He himself therefore devised new machines for both radium and high-voltage therapy. In the summer of 1933 he sailed for Europe to acquaint himself with the latest in radium "bombs," or devices containing several grams of radium. In Stockholm he placed an order for a special teleradium device of the kind designed by Swedish physicist Rolf Sievert ("teleradium" means a radium source at a distance from the body). It was a "bomb" consisting of 40 tubes, each containing 100 milligrams of radium. TGH engineer Albert Darbyshire then fashioned a curved track along which the device could travel so that the rays would always be focused at a precise spot beneath the skin without subjecting the intervening tissue to too much damage. This was considered to be the first of its kind in North America and it began service at the Institute in March 1934.[33] (The Ministry of Health rented the radium for the bomb, as opposed to its usual policy of purchasing radium from a Belgian firm and from the Canadian company Eldorado Gold Mines.[34])

Second, Richards pressed forward with more powerful super-volt therapy than offered by the two 200 kV machines already on hand. Together with technologists Tommy Hurst and Arthur F. Jeans, Richards designed a 400 kV unit with a space for the patient (who had to remain motionless in front of the tube for up to forty minutes) resembling a small hotel room. ("The patient's comfort is our primary aim," said Richards.) The TGH trustees and Richards had gone directly to the premier of the province to appeal for funds,[35] and it was with a grant from the Ontario government that the Picker X-ray Company of Toronto was able to build it. The machine came into use in 1937. It was soon enlarged to permit the treatment of four patients at once. There were 600 pounds of lead in the door of each apartment. Again, the machine was said to be a first for North America.[36]

The care Richards took in making the machine congenial to patients illustrates a larger point: Despite his reputation for gruffness, he was usually at great pains not to add unnecessarily to the suffering of his patients. In treating breast cancer patients post-operatively, for example, he originally made a plaster cast of the patient's chest wall, fitted the radium needles in the mold, and had the patient wear it about. Then he determined that a jacket-style cotton cover for the chest would be more comfortable, and placed the needles in that. In treating cervical cancer the fashion was to insert the metal radium applicators into the cervix in a casing of rubber. This was stiff and uncomfortable. Just as nylon was coming into style in the late 1930s, he tried encasing the applicators in nylon moulds. "Because women are not all the same size," as his biographer explained, "he made applicators in four sizes. These… were much more comfortable for the patient."[37] This attentiveness to his patients' well-being did not go unnoticed. In the mid-1940s about a hundred women whom Richards had treated for breast cancer—all 5 to 17 year "cures"—organized a dinner in his honor. "It was a very happy occasion and after the formal part was over the women all had a chance to chat with the man who had prolonged their lives and given them new hope." As for Richards, states his biographer: "[It] made him feel that the struggles and disappointments of his profession were not important when compared to the rewards."[38]

Radium, supervolt therapy: these were such noble initiatives, who could be against them? Through this period runs an undercurrent of hostility from the surgeons, who saw radiation oncology as eating away at their patient base. When in 1934 the provincial government set up a cancer committee, "The minutes record that the expenditures of the Government on radium encountered considerable opposition from some of the surgeons in attendance…."[39] (The opposition could not have been too embittered, for afterwards all dined at the Ontario Club, yet the behind-the-scenes note was clear.) An undated cartoon of the 1930s from an undergraduate medical student publication shows Richards and TGH chief surgeon William E. Gallie struggling over a patient. It was a struggle the surgeons generally won: In 1948 sixty percent of the 1800 new cancer cases seen at TGH were still treated with surgery alone, 30 percent with radiation, and only 10 percent with combined therapy.[40]

As a footnote it might be remarked that this problem was not resolved even under the Ontario Cancer Institute. The executives of the Ontario Cancer Treatment and Research Foundation who were planning the Ontario Cancer Institute in the mid-1950s somewhat lamely dismissed any responsibility for including surgery in their program: "No attempt has been made to centralize the surgical treatment of cancers in the therapy centres of the Foundation." They explained, however, that they might send out radiotherapists to consult with the surgeons at referring hospitals. This would be "to carry on joint follow-up examinations and to discuss the problems of combined and planned therapy of cancer."[41] Right into the 1990s the OCI found it difficult to offer comprehensive care to cancer patients because of the surgeons' fear of losing business. Said one radiation oncologist in 1994: "We still don't have a comprehensive surgical oncology division in the 1990s.... The surgeons felt they were going to lose patients completely to PMH, although in fact they never did."[42]

Under Richards in the late 1930s, the Ontario Institute of Radiotherapy became a world-center of cancer therapy. Richards had perfected techniques for treating cancers of the lip and tongue, and the message the Institute was putting out to the public was that early treatment could mean the curability of many other cancers too.[43]

In his later years Richards became the acknowledged leader of radiation oncology in Canada. In 1943 he helped found the Ontario Cancer Treatment and Research Foundation (OCTRF), becoming its first managing director. (The story goes that he was so indignant at the efforts of the Ontario government to siphon funds from the TGH cancer clinic to the other provincial clinics that he appealed to the cancer committee of the Ontario Medical Association, and became reconciled only by receiving the post at OCTRF.[44]) In 1938 Richards helped found the Canadian Cancer Society. His fundraising efforts in 1946 permitted the Ontario branch of this society to establish a permanent office. In 1947 he and Allan Blair organized the National Cancer Institute. Richards became its first president in 1948, a year before his death of leukemia.[45] At his death the trustees of the Toronto General Hospital noted with pride that Richards had introduced high-voltage therapy to Canada, that he had safeguarded the "first adequate supply of radium" in the land, and that he had developed "the first great Radium Bomb—all three were pioneered at this Hospital."[46] In the history of cancer therapy in Canada, Gordon Richards' contributions were monumental. In the judgment of his distinguished contemporary, the physicist Harold Johns, it was Richards' stature that "made Canada a leader in radiotherapy."[47]

The Ash Years

In radiotherapy, demand constantly expands to meet supply. Despite the creation of the six other provincial cancer clinics and the Ontario Institute of Radiotherapy at TGH, the backlog of patients seeking treatment continued to lengthen. By 1944 it had become so long that some of them were dying before receiving treatment. Early in the war the Toronto clinic recommended to the province that the number of beds at its disposal be increased from fifty to a hundred. The Minister of Health replied that one possibility might be establishing a free-standing cancer hospital independent of the city's general hospitals. In 1944, the Toronto General Hospital viewed this prospect with some misgiving.[48]

In 1944 Clifford Ash was thirty-five years old. Ash, who would take the baton from Richards as Toronto's chief radiotherapist, was a westerner. Born in 1909 in Edmonton, he did his BSc at the University of Alberta and came to Toronto for his MD, which he earned in 1934. He worked summers to put himself through school, including a stint as "tent boy" for a Chautauqua travelling theater group. During his internship at the Toronto Western Hospital, he met a Major Shanks who had been in the Indian Medical Service. Ash and his classmate Lawson ("Scotty") MacCullough were soon convinced to sign up. In the fall of 1935 the two dashing young physicians (Ash had worked as a tennis instructor at a resort hotel in Huntsville owned by his fiancée's uncle) went to England to train in tropical diseases. Ash then returned at Christmas time, married Eleanor Sanson, and in April 1936 the young couple sailed

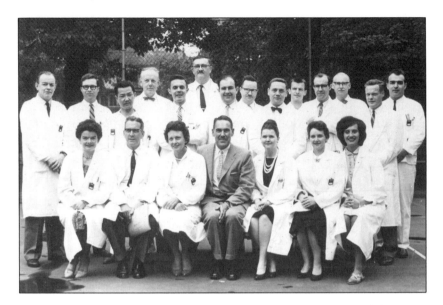

Figure 12. Princess Margaret Hospital staff, 1959. Harold Warwick, Vera Peters, and Clifford Ash are seated second, third, and fourth from the left. Bill Rider is standing at the far left, and the towering figure sixth from the left is John Darte.

back to England. Ash then spent the next two years at various posts of the Indian Medical Service, including the Indian Military Hospital in Bangalore and the St. Thomas' Hospital in Madras. This adventuresome period came to an end in 1938 as Ash developed tropical sprue and was invalided home.[49]

Between 1938 and 1940 Ash trained in radiology at the University of Toronto, qualifying for the diploma in that subject in 1940. Ash was essentially a student of Richards and was said to venerate the older man, whose background was so similar to his own.[50] Ash spent 1949 at various European centers with the aid of a British Empire Cancer Campaign Fellowship. Then in 1952, three years following Richards' death, he became head of the Ontario Institute of Radiotherapy, which is to say, head of the therapeutic side of the radiology department of the Toronto General Hospital.

A rugged, handsome man, Ash had the reputation as being, in the recollection of colleague Bernard Shapiro, "the nicest mildest human being you ever met." He remained youthful in appearance. When Bernard Shapiro was a candidate for the Royal College fellowship exam, he happened to meet Ash in the antechamber. In the belief that Ash was also a candidate, Shapiro started joking around, "If they want to know how to treat breast cancer I can tell them how Richards does it, and how somebody else does it, and when I walked in [there was Ash sitting down as an examiner].

"He said to me, 'So which therapy for carcinoma of the breast are you going to tell me about' and I almost died. I got so excited. The other examiner said, 'You better have a cup of tea, you look sort of pale.' Cliff Ash was a real nice man."[51]

Colleague Günes Ege remembered Ash as "kindly, imposing physically, large, yet warm and soft." "He was very much a father figure."[52] And just as Richards had once gone down to the General on Christmas Day to carve the turkey for the cancer patients, so did Ash put on his morning suit at eleven "and go around to his patients' bedside and serve them their Christmas dinner," as his daughter Judith recalled. "He'd come home around one or two and then we would have our Christmas dinner after that."[53]

In 1951 the Ontario government announced that it would be creating a big new cancer clinic, ultimately named the Ontario Cancer Institute. The OCI was the administrative framework of a cancer therapy program that from 1958 on would be housed in its own independent hospital, the Princess Margaret Hospital, and funded by the Ontario Cancer Treatment and Research Foundation (which in turn was funded by the province). Singleton was acting director until Ash was appointed director in July 1952. In 1956 Ash would give up his busy private radiotherapy practice in the Medical Arts Building to devote full-time to running OCI (OCI did not physically exist until the radiotherapy staff at TGH moved into the Princess Margaret Hospital in 1958).

Why this big new cancer initiative? Driving the idea of a separate cancer hospital in Toronto was a tremendous increase in rates of cancer in Ontario. Between 1934 and 1958 cancer death rates increased 86 percent for males and 48 percent for females. Particularly striking was the rising rate of lung cancer in males, which had risen almost five-fold.[54] For the OCTRF in 1950, the causes of this increase in lung cancer were a mystery: "In this series it was impossible to determine what factors might have been responsible for the change."[55] Yet the need for increased radiotherapy facilities was undeniable.

Early in 1945, Arthur Ford, the publisher of the *London Free Press* and chairman of the OCTRF, told E. C. Fox, chairman of the board of the Toronto General Hospital, that "this Hospital will likely be called on at an early date to make plans for the building and maintenance of a cancer unit containing 100 free beds."[56] TGH was quite pleased at the notion of being chosen as the site of a big provincial cancer hospital and at the corresponding expansion of its own influence. There was in the late 1940s no suggestion that the new cancer institute would be independent of TGH.[57] In 1949 a committee of university presidents chaired by Sidney Smith, president of the University of Toronto, recommended that a "Toronto Institute of Radiotherapy" be established at the Toronto General Hospital. Other teaching hospitals would, however, share in the facility, so that "any suggestion of monopoly by the Toronto General Hospital would be overcome."[58] The new institute might be situated in or near the Wellesley Hospital (then a part of TGH) but the understanding was that TGH would run the show.[59]

In January 1951, following a brief from the Ontario Cancer Treatment and Research Foundation, Premier Leslie Frost proposed the establishment of an Ontario Cancer Institute to be situated in the Wellesley Division of TGH.[60] Then in June the picture changed dramatically for radiology at the General. Apparently in response to protests from the other hospitals, Frost determined that the new cancer hospital would have a board of trustees of its own, and that only two of the eight seats would belong to TGH. The TGH trustees went along with this, apparently mollified by the suggestion that the chairman of the cancer hospital board would be the chairman of the board of TGH (yet this was never realized).[61]

When the Cancer Act of 1952 renamed the institute the Ontario Cancer Institute, the penny finally dropped for the medical staff of the General Hospital: They had lost control of the province's radiotherapy program.[62] But the new quarters would not be ready for another few years, and in the meantime the OCTRF was willing to pay for a handsome new expansion of radiotherapy at the Toronto General Hospital.[63]

To be sure, TGH's was not the only cancer therapy program in town. In the early 1920s the Hospital for Sick Children offered x-ray treatment of eczema and ringworm of the scalp, and late in the 1920s would begin radium-plaque therapy for skin cancer.[64] HSC had readily acquiesced in 1950 to the creation of a new cancer hospital.[65] Although the children's hospital had toyed in the 1950s with the idea of running a substantial cancer clinic, William Cosbie at the OCTRF finally told them this was not on, and as PMH opened in 1958 they reached a compromise: children over 18 months would been seen at the Princess Margaret Hospital; those under 18 months would be treated at the Toronto General Hospital and followed up at the Hospital for Sick Children.[66]

The other teaching hospitals were never really players in the radiotherapy area. The minor radiotherapy programs available in the 1950s at the Mt. Sinai Hospital and St. Michael's Hospital folded after Princess Margaret Hospital opened, or as in the case of the tumor clinic at Sunnybrook Hospital, became outposts serviced by clinicians sent up from PMH.

In the 1950s radiation oncology meant Clifford Ash's program at the Toronto General Hospital. Ash set out to recruit the best radiotherapists in the world, who were at that time British. Because of his fellowship year in the United Kingdom in 1949, he knew many of them already, and proceeded to bring them over to the radiotherapy division of the Toronto General Hospital, until the Princess Margaret Hospital should be ready.

In February 1956 Ash brought over William Allt from the Meyerstein Institute of Radiotherapy of the Middlesex Hospital in London, where he had been an assistant radiotherapist for the previous four years. Allt was then thirty-seven. He had graduated in medicine from Dublin in 1943 and became interested in radiology in the last two months that he spent as a medical officer in the

Royal Navy at the end of the war. (Someone had asked him to take charge of an x-ray service, which he then knew nothing about.[67]) He trained in radium therapy at the Middlesex Hospital and the Mount Vernon Hospital and Radium Institute in Northwood, a branch of the Middlesex. In Toronto he would specialize in super-voltage therapy, especially of gynecologic cancers.[68]

Next in this wave of English and Irish radiotherapists came Walter D. ("Bill") Rider. Born around 1923, Rider grew up in Darlington, England, in a family line of veterinarians. He wanted to be a vet too, but his father told him, at a time when many vets were unemployed during the Depression, "Either you become a butcher or a doctor. You never see a thin butcher or an out-of-work doctor." Rider graduated in 1945 in medicine from Edinburgh. "With itchy feet," as he put it, he took a year off and did a residency year in Virginia, travelling as well to Canada. He then returned to the University of Edinburgh and trained in radiotherapy from 1948 to 1954 at the Edinburgh Royal Infirmary, receiving a staff appointment in 1954. Although Rider had disliked Toronto on his first visit, in 1956 he was willing to accept Ash's arguments that his future lay at the Ontario Cancer Institute. "It wasn't just the thought of working at the new hospital," he told a journalist. "It was the team that Clifford Ash had put together that, more than anything, changed my mind about Toronto."[69]

Rider was already well-known for a 1955 paper on multiple myeloma, the first clinical report on combination chemotherapy in the literature. He would later initiate at Princess Margaret Hospital total body and half-body radiotherapy, and was said to be the originator of the Toronto approach to radiotherapy, which meant irradiating tumors first and reserving surgery for failure. In cancer of the larynx he promoted radiation instead of surgery as a way of saving the patient's power of speech. He became the head of radiation oncology at Princess Margaret Hospital and in 1986 received the Gold Medal of the American Society for Therapeutic Radiology and Oncology, the greatest recognition that a North American radiation oncologist can achieve.[70]

Among Ash's recruits there was a singular catch from internal medicine: O. Harold Warwick. (The "O" stood for Orlando.) Born in 1915, Warwick obtained undergraduate degrees in Arts from Mount Allison University in 1936 and from Oxford in 1938 as a Rhodes Scholar. He graduated MD from McGill in 1940, the Gold Medalist of his class, and returned to England between 1941 and 1945 as a squadron leader in the Royal Canadian Air Force. Warwick did a residency at the Royal Victoria Hospital, then returned to England as a Nuffield Fellow at the Royal Cancer Hospital (later the Royal Marsden Hospital) and the Chester Beatty Institute under Professor Alexander Haddow, gaining his MRCP in London in 1947. Here he revived the interest he had developed as an undergraduate at Oxford in cell respiration and in ways of influencing cancer chemotherapeutically. While in England he co-authored one of the early papers on nitrogen mustard therapy in the treatment of lung cancer.[71] (The very first papers on chemotherapy had started to appear in 1946 from Chicago). In 1947 he returned to McGill with a staff post in internal medicine at the Royal Vic.[72]

Then Warwick was summoned to Toronto to be a cancer executive, serving from 1948 to 1955 as the joint executive director of the National Cancer Institute of Canada and the Canadian Cancer Society. He also headed a ward in the Department of Medicine at TGH and was, in effect, the first medical oncologist in Canada. As head of TGH's Committee on the Chemotherapy of Cancer (and as OCI's senior physician), he and internist K. J. R. ("Kager") Wightman began using variants of nitrogen mustard that he received from colleagues in Britain in the treatment of lymphoblastomas.[73] In August 1955 he joined the radiology department of the General as a consultant in medical oncology. Shortly after moving to PMH, in 1959 Warwick would be first in North America to give the early vinca alkaloids to patients.[74] Later in life this gifted and scholarly man became Dean of Medicine at the University of Western Ontario.

Two other names rounded out this powerhouse in radiotherapy that Ash was assembling at the General in the mid-1950s. Both were Canadians. Ironically, the one, a woman who had never set foot in the British Isles (at least professionally), was to become the most distinguished radiation oncologist of all.

John Darte was born in 1920 in Welland, Ontario, and graduated MD from the University of Toronto in 1944. After interning at St. Michael's Hospital he served in the Royal Canadian Air Force. Once demobilized in 1947 he was a resident first at St. Michael's in medicine, then at HSC from 1948 to 1950. By this time he was firmly directed toward pediatric hematology. In the 1950s he held a number of cancer appointments in Toronto, and fellowed several times in England, in 1956 as the Gordon Richards Fellow. In 1957 Ash brought him to the radiotherapy service of TGH as a "voluntary assistant," just before the transition to the Princess Margaret Hospital. Described a "a great mountain of a man with a kindly face and jovial smile,"[75] Darte dominated the field of pediatric hematology and pediatric radiotherapy in Ontario. In 1962 he would return from PMH to Sick Kids as the chief of hematology. At the time that his life ended suddenly three days after Christmas 1975 of a ruptured aortic aneurysm, he had again returned to PMH as chief radiotherapist.

The second was Vera Peters.

Vera Peters

The Toronto name with most historic resonance in the radiotherapy of cancer is that of Vera Peters. Ash did not recruit Vera Peters. He inherited her. Ash himself and Peters were Gordon Richards' only students who became prominent figures in radiotherapy in Toronto. And Vera Peters went on to acquire a place in the history of medicine that few other Toronto graduates have surpassed.

Mildred Vera Peters was born April 28, 1911, in a little farmhouse in what is now the Toronto suburb of Rexdale. Her father Charles Peters had inherited the farm from his parents. Her mother Rebecca ("Nellie") Mair was a schoolteacher. The first vehicle she learned how to drive was a tractor. She attended school in a

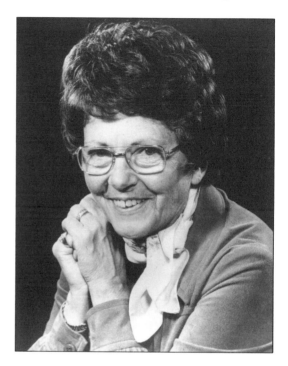

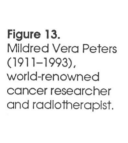

Figure 13.
Mildred Vera Peters
(1911–1993),
world-renowned
cancer researcher
and radiotherapist.

one-room schoolhouse in Thistletown. "She did all the grades as fast as you can," her daughter Jennifer Ingram later said. "She was very bright."[76]

Sixteen at graduation from high school, Peters was too young to qualify for medicine. So she entered U of T "via the backdoor" as a student in mathematics and physics. The following year she transferred into medicine hoping that no one would notice her age. No one did.

After graduating in medicine from the University of Toronto in 1934, she spent a year as a surgical resident at St. John's Hospital on Major Street in Toronto. At that point her mother was diagnosed with breast cancer and sought treatment from Gordon Richards, who put her into one of the radium jackets he had designed. Vera Peters, of course, was mindful of the long history of cancer in her family tree. When she met Richards in 1935 she became inspired by him and decided to do a kind of apprenticeship with him in radiotherapy, even though no formal program in the subject then existed in Toronto.[77] In the words of her memorialist Peter Fitzpatrick, "Dr. Richards became her mentor and he trusted her more than the other physician assistants. She learned to both love him and hate him at the same time and credits him for stimulating her interest in clinical observation, the importance of accuracy and the subsequent review of the medical record."[78] In April 1937 she was appointed "junior assistant radiologist" at TGH.[79] The Royal College "grandmothered" her into certification in radiation therapy in 1945.

In 1947 Richards assigned Peters the job of checking all his records of patients with Hodgkin's Disease. Said Peters later, "He asked if I would undertake a review of our past experience, to determine if anything was being accomplished by treatment. He had begun to sincerely doubt the incurability of the disease—some patients followed more than 10 years seemed to be cured!

"In spite of the then prevailing medical mood of despair, Dr. Richards believed in aggressive palliation. For patients presenting with large lymphatic masses, commonly neck or mediastinum, it was his policy to administer local radiation until the mass disappeared, or until the maximum tolerance of normal tissues in the radiated area had been reached."[80]

Following the practice of Geneva radiotherapist René Gilbert, Richards and Peters also radiated lymph nodes in nearby regions that were apparently healthy.

"Analyzing the 257 cases under review," said Peters, "turned out to be a monumental task." Peters would do her clinical work during the day but, as one chronicler of these events put it, "every night [she] carried home a sheaf of records for analysis. Evenings and weekends were spent gathering all the information into neat tables under different headings. Then she plotted the results on huge three-by-two foot graph paper." In January 1949 she reported at departmental rounds on 113 of the 257 Hodgkin's patients whom Richards had treated over the past twenty years (the others having been omitted because of lack of data or disagreements over diagnosis). Her large charts told the story: Among Richards' patients the five-year survival rate had doubled, the 10-year rate tripled.[81] The kind of aggressive radiotherapy used in Toronto after the

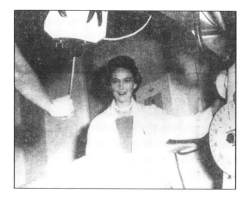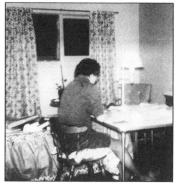

Figures 14 and 15. Vera Peters did her clinical work during the day... and spent her evenings and weekends at home analyzing case records by hand and plotting the results on huge sheets of paper.

muscular new machines arrived in 1935 was paying off. This was big news: a quarter of the patients with Hodgkin's Disease were being cured with radiation therapy.

A year after Richards died in 1949, Peters published these results, (essentially confirming that René Gilbert had been on the right track though she did not mention Gilbert's paper).[82] By building on Richards' work, Peters had established definitively that radiotherapy was a cure for a major cancer that previously was viewed as incurable. From these findings she worked out dosage and staging. (Staging is an important issue because the therapy selected may depend on the stage of the disease.) By 1957 her staging of Hodgkin's Disease had become the internationally accepted one.[83]

Peters' work was said to have galvanized Henry Kaplan of Stanford University to take on Hodgkin's Disease.[84] Kaplan, who became the most prominent American specialist, said many years later of Peters that she had "alerted the rest of the world" to the fact that radiating apparently healthy lymph nodes near the diseased nodes helped prevent the spread of the disease. By 1960 she was getting "the best results in the world" in treating Hodgkin's with radiation.[85]

Even before her involvement with Hodgkin's Disease Peters had been interested in breast cancer, doubtless owing to her mother's death from the disease. As early as 1944, the thirty-three-year-old "senior assistant" in the radiology department published a paper on the advantages of irradiating breast cancers before and after surgery.[86]

Because these were patients that she and Richards shared, next time it was he who published on the radiation therapy of breast cancer, and his 1948 paper—which fully acknowledged her help with statistics and with the construction of a clinical index of malignancy—emphasized even more strongly the advantages of radiation therapy in the management of breast cancer. Yet the paper did not challenge the need for radical mastectomy in the early stages. (In the later stages it was too late for radical mastectomy.[87])

TGH had a breast cancer clinic in which the radiotherapists and surgeons collaborated. After Richards' death, Peters and Ash carried on alone in collaboration with surgeons Robert M. Janes (the professor of surgery) and Norman Delarue. By 1953 the group had assembled sufficient data to permit them to cast doubt upon the effectiveness of the radical Halsted mastectomy.[88] This was among the earliest breaches in a doctrine that had forced many women with breast cancer to undergo radical mastectomy unnecessarily.

As Peters became known as a specialist in this area who favored minimally invasive treatments (and who was also extremely good at giving patients psychological support), she got many advanced breast cases as referrals. Especially she got those women who refused to consent to mastectomy and were turfed to her by surgeons exasperated at the challenge to their authority. As her daughter Jenny Ingram later put it, "She acquired these patients without a planned arrangement. The surgeons would know there was a female radiotherapist who would take these patients off them. Here's somebody who will understand your point of view, because she's female."

So Peters would take such patients into her clinic and treat them with radiotherapy following lumpectomy. "She began," Ingram continued, "to think these women were doing very well. She began

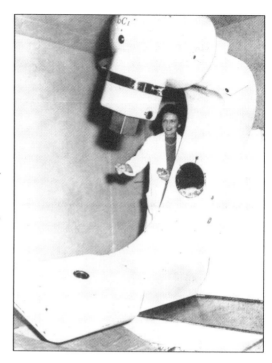

Figure 16.
Dr. M. Vera Peters at
the "Cobalt X-otron,"
the cobalt[60] beam
therapy unit disigned
by the scientific staff
of The Ontario Cancer
Institute. *Photo by
Cunningham, Gilbert
A. Milne & Co.* Ontario
Cancer Treatment
and Research
Foundation, *Annual
Report, 1958/59.*

to pull out files on the women who had lumpectomies and postop-
erative radiation, out of a gut feeling that they were doing well,
and started to age-match-control them for women diagnosed at the
same time who had radical surgery." The later paper she gave on
this created a sensation.[89]

Peters did her work on the dining-room table at night. Jennie
Ingram later said, "She had to be absolutely certain of her facts.
She was meticulous to a fault in how she matched her controls.
She categorized people by hand, and spent hours each night with
the dining-room table covered with patient files, great big nine-by-
sixteen sheets of paper with page after page of patients' names and
check marks for the type of class and how they did and where their
disease spread to."

Was she distracted by the racket of family life around her?
Ingram said, "When she got her thinking cap on, we used to kid
her. We would ask if we could commit suicide and she would nod
and say yes. She'd block everything else out. The story I always

tell about her was when she got in the car and had a cigarette—she smoked heavily—and threw the keys out the window into rush-hour traffic and stuffed the cigarette into the keyhole."

Did she pay a human price for this fast-paced research life? Ingram felt that her mother combined these roles seamlessly. In those years, the 1950s, she was among the first to explore the "completely unwritten territory," as Ingram put it, of "integrating family life with professional life." She was among the first of the highly successful female-physician role models. She had met her husband, Ken Lobb, in 1937 while both of them were putting themselves through school by waiting tables on the SS Kingston, a tourist ship that conducted two-day cruises on Lake Ontario. He later became a high-school gym teacher and vice-principal. She was sensitive to the career gap between them. "Mom was conscious of the fact that it could become an issue, and she worked hard at being very feminine and supportive. She tended to underrate her accomplishments to people around her and never wanted any attention drawn to herself." She kept her maiden name for the profession and was "very Mrs. Lobb at home." "She encouraged friends to call her Mrs. Lobb. The Dr. Peters character happened when she got into her car or arrived at the doors of the hospital." Yet so successfully did she juggle the twin demands of home and career that Ingram, then herself a medical student (Ingram later became an internist and geriatrician), felt she could bring her female friends from medical school home to dispel the notion that "you couldn't possibly have kids, if you did they'd grow screwed up. Here was a regular family who had dinner.... Here was a brilliant woman who was fun to be with. Also, there was a sense that if you went through medicine you were either a jerk or perfect. And here was a woman we kidded about being so deep in thought that at times she let the ashes from her cigarettes roll off onto the floor and burned holes and left the coffee cup in the refrigerator. She was a little bit the absent-minded professor, and she loved having this as part of the humor of the family. For my friend who had no role models this was like coming to the recognition that it's possible."

Not only therefore was Peters a pioneer in scientific terms, she was in personal ones as well. She and her classmate Jessie Gray, Toronto's first female surgeon, were the initial female medical graduates from Toronto to display lifetimes of major achievement.

Peters' achievements were acknowledged later in life, though at first some of her findings met with stiff resistance. In 1975 she became a member of the Order of Canada (in 1978 an "officer"). In 1977 she received the medal of the Centre Antoine Béclère in Paris, the first woman and the first North American to be so honored. In 1979 the American Society for Therapeutic Radiology granted her their Gold Medal (making Toronto the only center ever to have three such gold medalists, Harold Johns and Bill Rider being the other two).

In 1958 Peters moved with the rest of the staff of the Ontario Cancer Institute from the Toronto General Hospital to the Princess Margaret Hospital. She retired in 1976 and consulted for a number of years in private practice. In 1993 Peters died of breast cancer in the Princess Margaret Hospital. The following year one of the new "academies" for Toronto's medical undergraduates—the one at the Women's College Hospital and Mt. Sinai Hospital—was named in her honor.

Diagnostic and Therapeutic Radiology Separate

Diagnostic and therapeutic radiology began to diverge after the Second World War. In 1948, the combined examination in diagnostic and therapeutic radiology that the Royal College of Physicians and Surgeons in Ottawa had introduced two years previously was divided, making it possible to be examined on therapeutic radiology alone after 1948 (the field was renamed radiation oncology in 1976).[90] In Toronto the two fields had separated in practice with the appointment of Arthur Singleton in the 1920s, for Singleton looked after the diagnostic side, Richards the therapeutic. In the Dunlap Building members of each field would have lunch separately.[91]

The schism between the two disciplines was formalized at the General in 1950, as the medical advisory board determined that diagnostic radiology would take over the Dunlap Building until the new centre block was ready (it opened in 1959). The therapeutic side would move to renovated space elsewhere (which turned out to be the South Block on Gerrard Street).[92] In 1953 residents in radiology ceased alternating between the diagnostic and therapeutic sides.[93] Indeed in 1953-54 hospital staff lists began to distinguish between the "Department of Radiology—Diagnostic," with Singleton as radiologist-in-chief, and the "Department of Radiotherapy" with Ash as radiotherapist-in-chief.[94] As William Cosbie, medical director of the OCTRF and a gynecologic oncologist, said in 1958, "The day is past when radiotherapy can remain merely in association with diagnostic radiology." It was time for the two disciplines to go their separate ways.[95]

Driving this division was the relentless technologic advance in both disciplines. So high-tech did both become that they could not be successfully pursued without the active collaboration of physicists. Richards was apparently the first Canadian radiologist to enlist the collaboration of a physicist. In 1932 he asked John Leitch, who had a master's in physics and had just come to the provincial Division of Industrial Hygiene, to calibrate the equipment, check the radium, and supervise the radon plant that was going into the Department of Physics. Several members of the physics department helped Richards out in the late '30s and '40s.[96] In 1947, John Brown became OCTRF's first full-time medical physicist[97] and he was joined by two others in the late 1940s and early '50s.

Toronto's big coup in the area of physics was Ash's successful recruiting of Harold Johns in 1956 to head the division of physics of the Ontario Cancer Institute (a division that would be folded into OCI's joint department of medical biophysics, established in 1958). Johns pioneered postwar advances in both modes of radiation therapy: multimegavoltage in the form of the "betatron," and radioactivity in the form of a "bomb" using the radioactive isotope cesium-60.

Born in West China in 1915, Johns earned his BA at McMaster University in Hamilton, Ontario, and his PhD in physics in 1939 at the University of Toronto. After the war broke out, Johns found himself doing the radiography of aircraft castings in western Canada. He also lectured in physics at the University of Alberta, which being relatively near Saskatoon, helps explain why he took an assistant professorship at the University of Saskatchewan in 1945. Meanwhile, the young Allan Blair had gone from the radiology department of Toronto General Hospital to become director of cancer services in Saskatoon. Blair realized that they needed a full-time physicist, and the university and the Saskatchewan Cancer Commission jointly agreed to hire Johns.[98]

In May 1946 Blair sent Johns on a research trip involving a stopover in Toronto. Richards invited Johns to attend a lecture series at the Toronto General Hospital by Professor William V. Mayneord of the Royal Cancer Hospital in London, England on the physics of radiotherapy, which included the use of a linear accelerator to obtain a beam of gamma rays (instead of passing high voltages through an x-ray tube). This was a betatron, which Mayneord had first seen used at the University of Illinois in Urbana.[99] The development piqued Johns' interest and he went back to Saskatoon to ask that a betatron be ordered.

Two years later, in 1948, Illinois physicists at the University of Chicago attempted to use their betatron on a graduate student in physics who had a brain tumor. This was the first therapeutic use of the betatron. The second was Johns' in 1949 in Saskatoon.[100]

In a completely separate development, it happened that in Chalk River, Ontario, Canada possessed the only atomic pile in the world capable of projecting a stream of neutrons on a substance in order to make it radioactive in a manner suitable for medical usage. Mayneord had spent the war years at Chalk River in a survey of possible isotopes that might be used in cancer therapy. It was Mayneord and a collaborator who "fingered"—as Harold Johns put it—cobalt-60.[101] Johns and others immediately realized that these radioactive isotopes, far cheaper and more powerful than radium, could revolutionize the treatment of cancer. In June 1949

Johns visited Chalk River, then asked the president of the University of Saskatchewan to order a supply of cobalt-60. Two years later the first cobalt-60 therapy unit was installed in Saskatoon (a second at the University of Western Ontario following close on its heels). Virtually simultaneously in the fall of 1951 the first patients were treated with cobalt-60 in Saskatoon and London, Ontario. In December 1951 Johns published news of their work in the journal *Nature*.[102]

Harold Johns was recruited to Toronto in 1956, thus guaranteeing the University of Toronto a major international figure. He came as the head of the physics department of the Ontario Cancer Institute, becoming in 1958 professor of physics and medical biophysics. At his retirement in 1980 he was a towering international figure in radiotherapy, author of a textbook used by diagnostic and therapy trainees and winner in 1973 of a Gairdner Foundation International Award.

In 1953 the radiology department of TGH had acquired a cobalt-60 unit of the style used at the University of Western Ontario. After the Princess Margaret Hospital opened in 1958, Toronto would have a 22-megavolt betatron as well. The cobalt unit was placed in the former building of the Hospital for Sick Children on College Street. A newspaper story about the unit's unveiling showed Ash standing next to the "cobalt bomb." The caption read "Ontario Institute of Radiotherapy Director is bomb's boss."[103]

Originally Ash had intended that the Toronto General Hospital would retain a sizable proportion of cancer patients.[104] Events did not work out like that. Although TGH kept several high-voltage machines, and Ash remained officially on staff, cancer radiotherapy in Toronto became centralized in the Princess Margaret Hospital. Its story after 1958 constitutes a separate narrative, yet before 1958 the tale of cancer therapy in Toronto lay embedded in the history of the radiology department of the University of Toronto and of the Toronto General Hospital.

Endnotes

[1] Arthur U. Desjardins, "The Status of Radiology in America," *JAMA*, 92 (Mar. 30, 1929), pp. 1035-39, quote p. 1035.

[2] W. G. Cosbie, "The Centralization of Cancer Services—How Far Should It Go?" *AJR*, 105 (1969), pp. 487-499, quote p. 487.

[3] "William Henry Beaufort Aikens, 1859-1924," *AJR*, 12 (1924), p. 490; on Aikens' life see also the obituary in the *CMAJ*, 14 (1924), p. 1132, and W. G. Cosbie, *The Toronto General Hospital, 1819-1965: A Chronicle* (Toronto: Macmillan, 1975), p. 186.

[4] W. H. B. Aiken, "Radium and Its Action in Connection with Certain Diseases of the Skin," *Canadian Practitioner and Review*, 34 (1909), pp. 739-746; with co-author F. C. Harrison, "Recent Observations on the Therapeutic Use of Radium," *ibid.*, 36 (1911), pp. 1-10.

[5] On Aikens' role in the American Radium Society see E. R. N. Grigg, *The Trail of the Invisible Light* (Springfield: Thomas, 1965), p. 218.

[6] "Radium as a Remedy," *Women's Saturday Night*, Jan. 17, 1914, p. 1.

[7] Cosbie, *Toronto General Hospital*, pp. 186-187.

[8] TGH MAB, Mar. 6, 1917, p. 5.

[9] On the cost and provenance of radium in these years see Stephen B. Dewing, *Modern Radiology in Historical Perspective* (Springfield: Thomas, 1962), p. 114.

[10] WGH MAB, Sept. 25, 1920, p. 27.

[11] In 1920 Richards requested that Dickson's salary be increased from $6000 to $9000 a year. TGH Trustees, May 19, 1920, p. 112.

[12] TGH MAB, Jan. 3, 1921.

[13] "Special Meeting of the Council of the Faculty of Medicine," Nov. 10, 1919, p. 115. University of Toronto Archives, A86-0027, box 18.

[14] TGH Trustees, Feb. 16, 1921, p. 135.

[15] TGH Trustees, May 18, 1921, p. 145. The donor was Mr. William Addie.

[16] TGH Trustees, June 15, p. 147; Sept. 21, 1921, p. 184.

[17] TGH Trustees, Dec. 21, 1921, pp. 161-162. On the arrival of radium at TGH see also *Report of the Royal Commission on the Use of Radium and X-Rays in the Treatment of the Sick* (Legislative Assembly of Ontario, Sessional Paper no. 41, 1932) (Toronto: Ball, 1932), p. 11.

[18] "X-Ray Reveals Mysteries...," *Toronto Daily Star*, Nov. 15, 1924, p. 2.

[19] "First Radium Cancer Clinic at TGH," *Alumnae Association, School of Nursing, Toronto General Hospital, The Quarterly*, Fall, 1980, p. 1.

[20] On the acquisition of high-voltage machinery in the 1920s, see *Royal Commission on Radium*, p. 11.

[21] TGH Trustees, Sept. 28, 1927, p. 400. "The results of operation in the Department of Radiology would account for the total net loss in the operation of the Hospital."

[22] Gordon E. Richards, "Possibilities of Roentgen-Ray Treatment in Cancer of the Pancreas," *AJR*, 9 (1922), pp. 150-152, case p. 151. For a review of the literature giving Richards priority see George T. Pack and Gordon McNeer, "Radiation Treatment of Pancreatic Cancer," *AJR*, 40 (1938), pp. 708-714.

[23] Gordon E. Richards, "X-Rays and Radium in the Management of Breast Carcinoma," *CMAJ*, 16 (1926), pp. 358-366, quote p. 366.

[24] *Royal Commission on Radium*, p. 12.

[25] TGH Trustees, Nov. 24, 1926, p. 361.

[26] TGH MAB, Mar. 20, 1930, p. 25.

[27]TGH Trustees, Sept. 24, 1930, pp. 534-535.

[28]*Royal Commission on Radium*, p. 110.

[29]Summary of a talk Herbert Bruce gave at the Academy of Medicine, *Saturday Night*, Mar. 2, 1929, p. 1.

[30]*Royal Commission on Radium*, p. 15.

[31]*Royal Commission on Radium*, p. 101.

[32]On these events see TGH Trustees, Nov. 23, 1932; Mar. 22, 1933; Nov. 22, 1933; Mar. 28, 1934.

[33]Sources on Richards' teleradium bomb include "Toronto Doctor's Discovery," *Telegram*, June 4, 1935; Margaret Mason Shaw, manuscript "Gordon Richards," ch. 8, p, 2; Ontario Institute of Radiotherapy, Toronto General Hospital, *Sixth Annual Report, Year 1939* (Toronto: University of Toronto Press, 1940), p. 17.

[34]A. H. Sellers and J. H. Broughton, MS. "A History of the Ontario Cancer Treatment and Research Foundation" (1979), p. 29 and tabl. I. The OCTRF kindly made the manuscript available to the author.

[35]TGH Trustees, Oct. 28, 1936, p. 978. The minutes of Sept. 22, 1937, record that the premier authorized $35,000 for the supervoltage machine and the renovation of space.

[36]For details see *Toronto Daily Star*, Mar. 26, 1938, p. 7; Ontario Institute of Radiotherapy, *Sixth Annual Report*, pp. 26-29.

[37]Shaw, "Richards," ch. 6, p. 1.

[38]Shaw, "Richards," ch. 5, p. 6.

[39]As recalled in Norman McCormick to Ash, Nov. 29, 1956; I have this document from the Ash Family Papers owing to the kindness of Dr. Judith Ash.

[40]Harold Wookey, "The Ideal Coordination of Cancer Therapy," OCTRF, *Annual Report*, 1949, pp. 47-48, see p. 47.

[41]OCTRF, *Annual Report*, 1955, p. 34.

[42]Ege interview.

[43]See the series of articles by Richards in the *CMAJ*: "The Radiological Treatment of Cancer: Methods and Results, 1928-1935," vol. 35 (1936), pt. 1, "The Biological Conception of Dosage in Radiotherapy," pp. 299-305; pt. 2, "Carcinoma Cervicis Uteri" (with W. G. Cosbie), pp. 381-385; pt. 3, "Malignant Lesions of the Tonsil, and its Pillars," pp. 385-390; pt. 4, "Carcinoma of the Lips," pp. 490-502; pt. 5, "Carcinoma of the Tongue," pp. 593-603; pt. 6, "Intra-Oral Lesions (Except the Tongue)," pp. 599-603. On the OIR's message to the public see "Early Action in Cancer Held Essential Need," *Globe and Mail*, May 18, 1940.

[44]See McCormick to Cosbie, Nov. 29, 1956.

[45]On these efforts see the manuscript of a speech Clifford Ash gave to the OCTRF around 1975, pp. 4, 10. Ash Family Papers.

[46]TGH Trustees, Feb. 2, 1949, p. 1633.

[47]Harold E. Johns, "Impact of Physics on Therapeutic and Diagnostic Radiology," *JCAR*, 30 (1979), pp. 192-201, quote p. 194.

[48]TGH Trustees, "Toronto General Hospital Chairman's Report," May 3, 1944, pp. 8-9.

[49]On the years of his internship and Indian service see Eleanor Sanson Ash, MS. "The Family Sanson" (1989), pp. 50-52, 65-71. Ash Family Papers.

[50]"Pioneer Cancer Fighter Retiring," *Toronto Star*, Dec. 28, 1974, p. F2. The journalist who wrote the story, Lotta Dempsey, was doubtless well-informed of these matters as she was married to Ash's colleague, Arthur Ham.

[51]Bernard Shapiro interview, Jan. 24, 1995.

[52]Günes Ege interview, Nov. 15, 1994.

[53]Judith Ash interview, Nov. 28, 1994.

[54]OCTRF, *Annual Report, 1959-60,* pp. 46, 50.

[55]OCTRF, *Annual Report, 1950,* p. 16. The organization did note, however, that some authorities had incriminated "excessive and prolonged cigarette smoking."

[56]TGH Trustees, "Chairman's Report," May 2, 1945, p. 9.

[57]See TGH Trustees, Nov. 3, 1948, p. 1617; TGH MAB, Dec. 9, 1948.

[58]See R. M. Janes's summary of the events of 1949 in TGH MAB, Feb. 24, 1953, pp. 1-2.

[59]See TGH Trustees, Mar. 7, 1951, p. 1778.

[60]Sellers and Broughton, "History of OCTRF," p. 122.

[61]TGH Trustees, June 28, 1951, pp. 1805-06.

[62]See TGH MAB, Feb. 24, 1953.

[63]TGH MAB, Jan. 6, 1954.

[64]HSC, *Annual Report, 1922,* p. 38; on H. A. Dixon's requests for radium for treatment of skin conditions see for example HSC MAB, Apr. 25, 1927.

[65]HSC MAB, Jan. 9, 1950.

[66]HSC MAB, undated report of the cancer committee in 1958.

[67]William Allt interview, Feb. 20, 1995.

[68]William E. C. Allt, "Supervoltage Treatment in Advanced Cancer of the Uterine Cervix," *CMAJ,* 100 (1969), pp. 792-797.

[69]"Cut Above the Rest," *Toronto Star,* Sept. 22, 1988, p. B3.

[70]Information on W. D. Rider from his biographical file in the Toronto Academy of Medicine collection, deposited in the Fisher Rare Book Library of the University of Toronto, and from several speeches commemorating Rider's accomplishments, Department of Radiation Oncology, Princess Margaret Hospital.

[71]E. Boyland et al. [incl. O. H. Warwick], "The Effects of Chloroethylamines on Tumours, with Special Reference to Bronchogenic Carcinoma," *British Journal of Cancer,* 2 (1948), pp. 17-29.

[72]Interview with O. Harold Warwick, Feb. 21, 1995.

[73]University of Toronto, Faculty of Medicine, *Report of the Dean,* 1949-50, p. 49.

[74]Warwick told the story in "The Beginnings of Vinca Alkaloids," *Cancer in Ontario, 1982* (Toronto: OCTRF, 1982), pp. 25-28.

[75]"Meet Dr. Darte," [HSC] *Paediatric Patter,* 7 (Oct., 1966), p. 2.

[76]Jennifer Ingram interview of May 6, 1994.

[77]Peters gave 1935 as the date of her earliest work with the radiotherapy of Hodgkin's disease. See M. V. Peters, "Pioneering in Hodgkin's Disease," OCTRF, *Cancer in Ontario, 1982* (OCTRF, Toronto), pp. 17-18.

[78]This account is based on the manuscript of Peter Fitzpatrick's obituary of Vera Peters, which is somewhat more extensive than the published version (*Clinical Oncology,* 6 [1994], p. 66), and on various family memoirs in the Peters Family Papers. See also the author's interview with Jennifer Ingram.

[79]TGH Trustees, Apr. 28, 1937.

[80]Undated manuscript of speech, Peters Family Papers.

[81]Margaret Mason Shaw, manuscript "Gordon Richards," ch. 9, pp. 2-3.

[82]M. Vera Peters, "A Study of Survivals in Hodgkin's Disease Treated Radiologically," *AJR* 63 (1950), pp. 299-311.

[83]See Clifford Ash, "Conference on Hodgkin's Disease," OCTRF, *Annual Report*, 1957-58, p. 71.

[84]Walter S. Ross, "They're Curing an 'Incurable' Cancer," *Reader's Digest*, Dec., 1969, pp. 125-131, esp. p. 128.

[85]"City Radiotherapist Praised," quotes Henry Kaplan's remarks during a meeting of the American Cancer Society in Toronto. *Globe and Mail*, May 8, 1976.

[86]M. Vera Peters, "Radiation Therapy of Carcinoma of the Breast," *CMAJ*, 51 (1944), pp. 335-343.

[87]Gordon E. Richards, "Mammary Cancer: The Place of Surgery and of Radiotherapy in its Management," *British Journal of Radiology*, NS, 21 (1948), pp. 109-127, 249-258.

[88]Clifford L. Ash, Vera Peters and Norman C. Delarue, "The Argument for Preoperative Radiation in the Treatment of Breast Cancer," *Surgery, Gynecology and Obstetrics*, 96 (1953), pp. 509-521.

[89]M. Vera Peters, "Cutting the 'Gordian Knot' in Early Breast Cancer," *Annals of the Royal College of Physicians and Surgeons of Canada*, 8 (1975), pp. 186-192.

[90]Personal communication from Jean McQuilliam, RCPS, Ottawa, Feb. 21, 1995.

[91]R. Brian Holmes interview, June 3, 1994.

[92]TGH MAB, Feb. 9, 1950.

[93]TGH MAB, Dec. 17, 1953. Residents were referred to as "senior internes."

[94]TGH Trustees, staff list interfiled in minutes for 1955, pp. 1965- 66.

[95]William G. Cosbie, "Gordon Richards and the Ontario Cancer Foundation," *JCAR*, 9 (1959), pp. 1-7, quote p. 7.

[96]Ash, OCTRF address, 1975.

[97]OCTRF, *Annual Report, 1947*, p. 8.

[98]On Harold Johns' role in the development of radiotherapy in Saskatchewan see C. Stuart Houston and Sylvia O. Fedoruk, "Saskatchewan's Role in Radiotherapy Research," *CMAJ*, 132 (1985), pp. 854-864.

[99]For other details in addition to the Houston-Fedoruk article, I am indebted to the manuscript "CARO Centennial Project," kindly placed at my disposal by Dr. Günes Ege.

[100]Grigg, *The Trail of the Invisible Light*, pp. 344-345.

[101]Harold E. Johns and T. A. Watson, "The Cobalt-60 Story," OCTRF, *Cancer in Ontario, 1982*, pp. 20-24, quote p. 20.

[102]Harold E. Johns et al., letter: "1,000-Curie Cobalt-60 Units for Radiation Therapy," *Nature*, 168 (Dec. 15, 1951), pp. 1035-36. For details of these events see "CARO Centennial."

[103]"Hope Cancer Cure Possible...," undated news clip from *Telegram*, sometime in Nov. 1953.

[104]See TGH MAB, Sept. 18, 1952; June 11, 1953.

Chapter Three

Hospitals

Toronto represented one of the greatest concentrations of radiology in North America. Rather than being centered in a single university hospital, the city's academic radiologists were distributed among eight separate teaching hospitals, each with its own traditions and jealous of its own prerogatives. This duplication of services had obvious disadvantages. Yet the university radiologists were able to develop such strength across the board precisely because the individual hospitals often cultivated different strengths. In the end, the diversity these hospitals offered collectively made Toronto perhaps stronger than a single university hospital would have done. This chapter examines the development of radiology in each of the eight hospitals. The following chapter follows the forging of this diversity into a single university-wide program of training residents. One bears in mind that until 1985 the radiologist-in-chief at the Toronto General Hospital was simultaneously the chair of the university department of radiology, and responsible for the university-wide program.

Toronto General Hospital

To put the growth of a century in context, between Richards' arrival in 1917 and the time of his death in 1949, the radiology department at TGH went from two radiologists, two technicians and a stenographer to approximately a hundred workers.[1] Yet of those hundred in 1949, there were only seven radiologists.[2] And among those seven only two were partners, Arthur Singleton and Mack Hall. They employed three therapeutic radiologists: Clifford Ash and Vera Peters who were already veterans, and Owen Millar, who had just returned from a year's radiotherapy fellowship in England. In addition in 1949 there were two junior diagnostic radiologists, Kenneth MacEwen, who had been a protegé of Singleton, and Delbert Wollin, fresh from the Montreal Neurological Institute as a neuroradiologist.

Forty years later in 1990 (just a year before the merger with the Toronto Western Hospital), therapeutic radiology had been cleaved off entirely. The four diagnostic radiologists at TGH had grown to eighteen, representing every subspecialty from ultrasound to interventional.[3] Physically, in 1983 the diagnostic department had expanded from its quarters in the Urquhart Wing, where it had taken the street floor in 1959, into new space in the Eaton Building with forty-two rooms given over to imaging. In 1949 the department was doing around 30,000 examinations a year, in 1990 203,000.[4] Mastering growth of this magnitude was possible only through strong leadership.

Arthur Singleton guided TGH through the first decade of growth from the time he became acting head in February 1949 until his retirement in June 1962 as chief at TGH and professor of radiology. The Singleton years were noteworthy for several events.

Although Singleton had not a great deal of interest in scholarly research and publication, he made radiologic history in 1949 by establishing that x-rays could be used to identify bodies mutilated in mass disasters. In September 1949 the Great Lakes liner "Noronic" caught fire while on a cruise, creating a blazing inferno in which 119 of her 527 passengers perished, most of them suffocated in their state rooms, their bodies then charred in the blaze. A team led by Singleton and TGH technician Tommy Hurst was able to set up three mobile x-ray units in the Horticultural Building of the Canadian National Exhibition, which served as a temporary morgue. The team attempted to match x-ray films taken postmortem with antemortem plates of the victims secured by the Red Cross. By zeroing in on congenital bony anomalies, within ten weeks' time the team was able to identify 24 of the 35 individuals for whom films had been submitted.[5] The research became a classic in the identification of disaster victims and aroused widespread local attention as well.[6]

Not only did Singleton set up Ontario's first training course for radiographers, in the training of radiologists as well he was a key national figure. Under Singleton at TGH in the 1950s, a whole generation of Canadian radiologists got their start. It was said at the time of his death in 1968 that he had helped train about 25 percent of the country's practicing radiologists.[7] These achievements were recognized in 1957 as he became president of the American College of Radiology, and gold medalist of the Radiological Society of North America in 1962.

Yet behind the scenes the Singleton years were marked by scientific drift and a preoccupation with private practice. As one junior radiologist in Singleton's employ later said, "Arthur was mainly interested in the office in the Medical Arts Building. He was up there mornings, came to the General at noon for lunch, ran the department there for a couple of hours, then back up to the other place."[8] Meanwhile Mack Hall was actually in charge at the General until Singleton retired, after which Hall's center of gravity too shifted to the private offices on Bloor Street.

In 1959 Singleton had five other practices in Ontario aside from the Toronto General Hospital and its affiliate private office in the Medical Arts Building. Junior radiologists on salary for the Singleton-Hall partnership read films for the Princess Margaret Hospital, the Royal Victoria in Barrie, the General-Marine in Collingwood, St. Andrew's in Midland and the nearby public hospital in Penetang, and the Smooth Rock Falls Hospital. Their total billings to the hospital system in that fiscal year were $237,000, which made them by far the highest-billing group in the province.[9] Singleton got juniors such as Ross Lobb to handle the "country run" and Lobb was said to "live behind the wheel of a car."[10] Edward Lansdown, then a resident at the General, also got roped into the country run. En route to places like Collingwood, Lansdown would ask himself, "Why am I doing this?"[11] (It was Singleton's involvement in private practice that disqualified him from membership in the US-based Association of University Radiologists. Instead, Holmes became the first Canadian member, after he had qualified by refusing in October 1962 to attend any further in the partners' private practice.)

Recognizing perhaps that the Singleton-Hall partnership was perhaps too much of a good thing, Norman Urquhart, chairman of the board of trustees of the Toronto General Hospital, tried to cut it back. In December 1948 he tried to persuade the board to alter what was then the Richards-Singleton-Hall contract.[12] The board wanted Singleton to operate radiology "as an integral part of the Hospital, and not as a separate enterprise." He would receive a salary as director.[13] Singleton reacted furiously, handing in his resignation four days after Christmas 1951 (which he then withdrew as the board agreed to negotiate).[14] Not until May 1953 was an agreement somewhat more favorable to the hospital finally reached.[15] Yet the atmosphere in the radiology department had been thoroughly poisoned, bewildering the junior radiologists and giving them a sense that research counted for little.[16] (In truth, there were years when the only publications coming out of the department were Vera Peters'.) Singleton at one point told the idealistic young Brian Holmes that (as Holmes recalled), "He was all for research, but he put out his hand and rubbed his fingers and said, 'It doesn't bring in that green stuff,'" meaning that research didn't pay its own way.[17] Only with Hall's retirement in 1965 did the junior radiologists become real partners.

Yet with the fading of the old regime, a piece of sociability in the life of the hospital fell away as well. For under the Richards-Singleton-Hall partnership the partners owned all the equipment and paid all the nurses, technicians and other support staff directly as employees. Having a distinctive sense of solidarity the hundred-odd employees of the partnership formed a social group, the "Radiantics Club." "It was a closely-knit group of people," said Holmes later. "They organized Christmas parties and Halloween parties and such. They used to organize a day to go to the ballpark, and the photographer had a fishing shack up near Newmarket and they'd have a picnic up near his place. It was a big part of the ambience of the department when I arrived and it went right back to the Richards days. Richards fostered it as a way of getting some

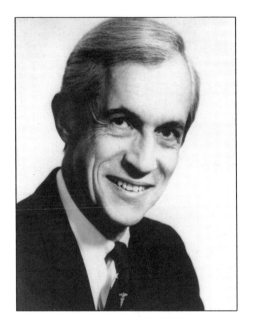

Figure 17.
Richard Brian Holmes.
His appointment as
chair of the university
department and
radiologist-in-chief at
Toronto General
Hospital in 1965
heralded the shift to a
new generation.

sense of a radiological community." The club went out of business around the time of Singleton's negotiations, because the hospital put all the support staff on salary.[18]

In 1965 Richard Brian Holmes was forty-five years old as he became professor and chairman of the university department of radiology and radiologist-in-chief at the Toronto General Hospital. It was time for the passing of the torch, and it was passed with a vengeance. Holmes was born in 1919 in London, Ontario, and became MD at the University of Western Ontario in 1943. After an internship at London's Victoria Hospital, Holmes took the Armed Forces Radiology Course at TGH and from 1944 to 1946 served as a radiologist in the Royal Canadian Army Medical Corps. He then became part of a growing postwar trend: seeking one's graduate training in the United States rather than in Britain. From 1947 to 1950 Holmes was a resident in radiology at the Massachusetts General Hospital in Boston, whence Singleton recruited him for Toronto in 1950.

With his leadership skills and overview of the field, Holmes became the leader of the Young Turks at TGH. Alongside him there were Delbert Wollin, six years Holmes's senior, who became so

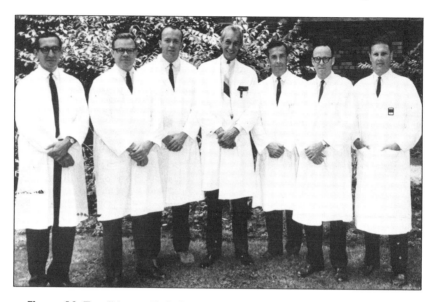

Figure 18. The "Young Turks" at TGH, 1965. Left to right: Ronald F.
Colapinto, Robert M. Parrish, Thomas H. Yates, R. Brian Holmes
(radiologist-in-chief), George Wortzman, Douglas E. Sanders, Edward
L. Lansdown.

alienated at the attitudes of the seniors that he left TGH for Calgary.
Kenneth MacEwen, MD from Toronto in 1939, had come to TGH
in 1947 and at the end of the 1950s would leave to become head
of radiology at the Wellesley Hospital. There was Ross Lobb, who
had grown up in Saskatchewan and was an exact contemporary of
Holmes's. Both graduated MD in 1943; both trained in radiology
during the war. Lobb came to the General in the mid-1950s.
Youngest of the group was Douglas Sanders, a University of
Toronto graduate who was thirty at the time of receiving his
fellowship from the Royal College in 1956. The age gap between
Singleton and Sanders was twenty-six years. So this clearly was a
new generation with very different ideas about science and the
importance of research in medicine.

Holmes lost no time in making clear that a new broom was
sweeping. "Until recently," he told his colleagues at the General,
"this Department was virtually unknown in international circles
because of the dearth of research and other scientific contributions
in the past. The staff member has tended to develop the conditional

reflex that unless he has reported a certain number of examinations per day... he has not carried out his share of the load." In consequence, any radiologist aspiring to be something more than a "reader of films" had experienced harassment. "A change in our thinking must occur if we are to establish a less hectic setting and replace it with one where some creative thinking can occur.... We must evolve from our rather parasitic role of only borrowing innovations from other centres and create our own small share of new ideas."[19]

This new sense of enthusiasm whirled into the office of Dean John Hamilton, who noted in his annual report that under the direction of Brian Holmes the radiology department had begun a major review of everything.[20] When he had been associate dean earlier, Hamilton seemed quite taken aback when Holmes pushed him about research: "I've never thought about research in connection with radiology," he told Holmes.[21]

Holmes had considerable initial success with his plan to get basic research going in radiology. But how was research to be paid for, given the paucity of funds made available by the university to the university department? To raise the $18,000 needed for the salary of the director, Holmes decided to cut the honorarium of the chairman of the university department to zero, then asked the Senior Committee to persuade department members to forego their annual teaching honoraria of $250. At Louis Harnick's motion, the committee agreed to contribute $200 for each department member, retaining only $50 per year, in Harnick's words, "to keep the mechanism open."[22] In 1971 the Radiological Research Laboratories were opened in the university's Medical Sciences Building, and Eric Milne, a well-known chest radiologist and scientist, was brought in to direct the unit.

Milne departed in 1975, when Holmes had already left the department and was dean of medicine. Yet after 1975 the laboratories did not fare well in terms of radiologic research and, even though radiologist Barry Hobbs was seconded from the TGH department to the laboratories several days a week, they became given over increasingly to physics. In 1981 the laboratories moved to the College Wing of the General, taking over space of the cardiovascular investigation unit that had been damaged by fire. Later, this group of researchers disappeared entirely from the General, and what little was done in Toronto in terms of basic research in radiology would take place at the Toronto Western Hospital and at Sunnybrook. (These are narratives that go beyond Holmes's tenure at the General, and will not be pursued here because they are marginal to the development of radiology in Toronto as a discipline.)

The challenges that Holmes faced were not all in the area of research. The department was expanding rapidly in the 1960s and by 1967 it included eight diagnostic radiologists and five voluntary assistants.[23] Office space had to be created for these newcomers. Holmes petitioned the trustees for a major physical expansion of the department. It was granted without caviling.[24] Two years later many of the hospital's big departments lay embroiled in strife around financial priorities. Again, radiology put its wish list through relatively untouched, which included air conditioning for the arteriography area, a new X-ray office, and renovations to the Burnside Building for nuclear medicine.[25] (It did not perhaps hurt matters that Holmes was interim chairman of the meeting of the medical advisory board that approved these priorities.) Such was the impact Holmes was making on the radiology scene in the late 1960s that a group of his former residents inaugurated a "Holmes Society," which would have an annual scientific meeting with invited guest lecturers.[26]

In scientific terms, the principal development at TGH in the 1960s was the rise of the radiologic subspecialties. Neuroradiology commenced at TGH in 1938 with the establishment of an encephalography unit in one of the operating rooms. This occurred six years after lumbar air encephalography was first described.[27] Douglas Eaglesham was TGH's first neuroradiologist. Like many high-profile physicians, Eaglesham came from a small town in the prairie provinces, in this case Saskatchewan. He graduated MD from the University of Manitoba in 1932, interned in radiology at the Royal Victoria Hospital in Montreal, then came to TGH in

1946. As Eaglesham moved on to Sunnybrook Hospital in 1947, Del Wollin replaced him. This was the heroic period of neuroradiology, when the radiologist was at the beck and call of the neurosurgeons. "If a patient came in with a subdural or brain tumor," recalled one of Wollin's associates, "the surgeon would see that patient and decide what needed to be done and then went home to bed. Wollin had to get out of his bed, come to the hospital and do it. And if the surgeon said, "This guy needs an arteriogram then a ventriculogram, the resident in neuro would do the arteriogram or put air into the ventricle, sedate the patient, and send him to the radiologist. Then somebody had to be there not only to watch the patient but to make sure the proper procedure was done. This was not for a technician. You had to have a radiologist. Some days I would come to work at eight and I would see Wollin going home. He'd been there all night."[28]

With Wollin's departure in 1959, George Wortzman became TGH's neuroradiologist. Wortzman had really followed in Eaglesham's footsteps. Born in 1924, Wortzman, like Eaglesham, had graduated MD from the University of Manitoba in 1950. After four years of general practice in Rivers, Manitoba, he had come east to train, again like Eaglesham, in radiology at the Royal Victoria Hospital in Montreal. At the time Montreal was Canada's most distinguished center of diagnostic radiology, and Wortzman learned neuroradiology from Donald McRae at the Montreal Neurological Institute. By 1959 Wortzman had probably become the best trained young neuroradiologist in Canada. He let himself be lured to the General. Wortzman went on to have a major international career and in 1980-81 was president of the American Society of Neuroradiology.

Holmes devoted much attention to bringing neuroradiology along, securing in the late 1960s large appropriations for a neuroradiographic unit and equipment for neurosurgical angiography.[29] Neuro was the first radiologic subspecialty to develop in Toronto and grew up along with neurosurgery. (Neurosurgeon Andrew Joachim was the first fellow in neuroradiology.[30])

The other subspecialty in which TGH pushed ahead was cardiovascular radiology, Holmes's own field. "Brian Holmes was the instigator of all the cardiovascular side," said a colleague in a later interview. "But he was not a person who dictated to anybody. He made suggestions diplomatically. He never offended anyone and made a point of initiating interest among people who were trying to learn."[31]

The major step in the development of the cardiac subspecialty was angiography. The field of angiography became transformed in the 1950s. First, in 1953 the Stockholm radiologist Sven Ivar Seldinger introduced the catheter named after him, a percutaneous flexible catheter.[32] This made it possible to gain access to individual blood vessels. In the same year, the first commercially-produced image amplifiers became available, harnessing TV technology to fluoroscopy. Radiologists no longer had to spend endless intervals adapting themselves to the dark and walk around in red glasses. Also, the new bright images could be recorded on film or videotape. At the opening ceremony in October 1960 of TGH's new "Marconi Image Orthicon," one radiologist told a reporter that, "He had seen more chalk in coronary arteries in the six weeks they had been using the machine than he had seen all the rest of his life as a radiologist."[33] Holmes used the motion-picture camera sold with the Image Orthicon to help introduce cineradiology to North America. He and resident Carmelle Thorfinnson published the first paper on cine-venography that showed the dynamics of the blood flow. They injected dye into the veins of patients with varicosities, filming the dye as it came up the leg, then watching as it refluxed at the site of the destroyed valves and flowed back down the leg to form an ulcer. Interpreting these moving pictures was far simpler than the previous static images.[34]

With image amplification in place, the development of a vascular, cardiac and chest subspecialities began in earnest.[35] Several enthusiastic young residents and junior staff moved into angiography. Douglas Sanders had a background in radiologic pathology at the Armed Forces Institute in Washington and had fellowed at

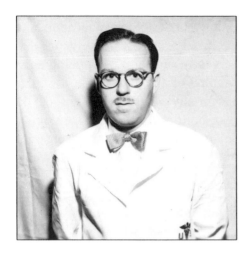

Figure 19.
Douglas E. Sanders, pioneer in angiography. With the Armed Forces Institute of Pathology, Washington, January, 1954.

Westminister Hospital in London, England. He was open to new ideas. "As that equipment became available," he said, "young guys that were in training or new staff radiologists like myself were thrust into it. In order to keep junior guys busy, they were told, 'You go and do that.' That's how I started."[36] In the late 1950s and early 1960s Sanders collaborated in several important papers on chest angiography to establish whether various lung cancers were operable.[37]

Another of the enthusiastic juniors was Ted Lansdown. His recollections of angiography went back to 1959, six years after Seldinger introduced his catheter. "When I first arrived at TGH I can remember they didn't have image intensification, and a catheter the size of a garden hose would be put up into the vessel by the new Seldinger Swedish technique. They'd turn out the lights, and as a resident one of my jobs was to take off my red goggles—everything in the room's dark—, climb up on the table and look through the old fluoroscopic machine and see where this radio-opaque catheter was in relation to the lumbar vertebrae. They'd turn on the lights and would inject some material and have an aortogram.

"Well, Ron Colapinto and I were the first ones to start angio with selective arteries, that is sticking catheters into specific smaller arteries."[38]

It was with image amplification that radiologists began to take angiography away from the surgeons. Previously the surgeons had done all the angiography themselves, the urologist the pyelograms, the chest surgeon the angiography of the lungs, the vascular surgeon the legs. They would essentially ask the radiologists to do no more than come and push the button. But as the radiologists gathered skill with the new technique, it no longer made sense for surgeons to continue to perform the procedure because the radiologists did many more of them and were more practiced. Thus in most centers angiography shifted away from surgery and towards radiology. This was true of every field save cardiology.

Brian Holmes was mindful of these trends. Around 1961 he said to Ronald Colapinto, then a senior resident, "Why doesn't radiology just do the whole procedure? Why don't you start doing it?" Colapinto, born in Toronto in 1931, had graduated from the University of Toronto in 1955. After a internship and a year of general practice, he decided to train in medicine at the University of Western Ontario, then in 1958 shifted to diagnostic radiology at TGH. It was in a fellowship year in 1961 that he and Holmes began working on coronary artery calcification, and in that context Holmes suggested angiography to him.

Colapinto proceeded to apply himself to angiography in an almost single-minded fashion... "We started reading books on 'how do you put a catheter in,'" he later said.[39] Holmes: "Colapinto was focused 110 percent on catheter work." In 1964 Colapinto had a fellowship to study angiography in Sweden, becoming director of the angiography division of TGH in 1967. It was Colapinto who got angiography going in Toronto, not just in the cardiac field but in many areas. His major achievements were to come in the late 1970s and after in the interventional area of creating shunts through the liver to relieve pressure in the portal circulation with the use of the "Colapinto" needle (see p. 162).

Image amplification was the first really high-tech device to hit diagnostic radiology, a field that until then had been confined to the reading of plain films and a bit of fluoroscopy. This technology was slow to come to TGH because Singleton kept insisting, as

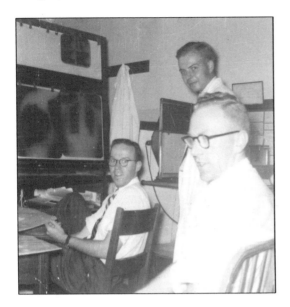

Figure 20.
TGH residents in radiology, at the Dunlap building, 1954: Sanders, Larry Mallett, and Kenneth Middlemiss.

Lansdown remembered his words, "We're training people to go out into the periphery and they won't have intensifiers." But Singleton delayed so long, Lansdown said, "that the periphery had them and we were the only ones that didn't." Once image amplification had established itself at TGH, there was no turning back. Although image amplifiers were hugely expensive, the board of trustees of the hospital did not blink at acquiring a second one in 1963 for the radiology department itself (the first had gone to the cardiovascular unit). The board found it no problem that the machine would cost $76,000 rather than the anticipated $50,000.[40] Driven forward by the hospital's vascular surgeons,[41] the General invested increasingly in image amplification, and the reputation of cardiovascular radiology grew with the reputation of cardiovascular surgery. Cardiovascular surgeon W. G. ("Bill") Bigelow, a pioneer in closed- and open-heart surgery, later acknowledged the support of radiology: "Guided by their special interest in the cardiovascular system, the Department of Radiology offered us all that was new in motion picture angiograms." "Brian Holmes, Chief of Radiology, Douglas Sanders, and Ronald Colapinto were responsible for providing our team with the finest in radiological

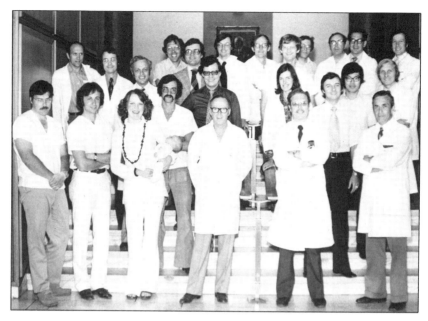

Figure 21. Toronto General Hospital. Radiology Department Staff, c. 1975. Douglas Sanders, Edward Lansdown, and George Wortzman are in the front row. Ronald Colapinto is second from right in the back row.

diagnosis at a time when the techniques were under constant change."[42]

In February 1972 Holmes stepped down from the chair of radiology to become associate dean of medicine (then dean of medicine in 1973-1980). For eighteen months Doug Sanders was acting chair, whereupon in 1974 Edward ("Ted") Lansdown returned from Manitoba to chair the radiology department at the General—and the university department as well—during a crucial decade of growth. Born in Winnipeg in 1927, Lansdown had graduated in medicine in 1957 from the University of Manitoba. He trained in radiology at TGH and the Hospital for Sick Children, then became a staff member of the department—with a specialty in cardiovascular research. In 1968 Lansdown returned to Winnipeg, first as a radiologist at the Winnipeg General Hospital, then from 1969 to 1974 as director of radiology at the St. Boniface General Hospital. In 1974 he came back to Toronto as chief at the General and professor of the department. The challenges that

Lansdown faced in the area of body imaging and unifying the training program are considered in later chapters. What assailed him from the very beginning, however, was ensuring that service in radiology at the General kept pace with the terrific growth the department was experiencing.

Service is a crucial question in radiology. The achilles heel of radiologists historically has been poor communication with referring physicians and tardiness in providing reports. Radiologist Richard Heilman at the University of Vermont once pointed out that the more sophisticated radiologic equipment becomes, the more dissatisfied grow the clinical consumers of radiologic services. "These insular subspecialists, operating without a comprehensive imaging plan and often provided with only a patient's name... generate reports that, when they are finally bound together (often in the medical-records department, days after discharge), constitute disorganized and imprecise documents that can rarely be taken seriously by clinicians."[43] Thus the more technologically complex the department grew, the greater would be the challenges Lansdown faced in delivering service to the rest of the hospital.

Holmes had tried to expand the availability of services in 1967 by bringing in a rapid-reading program, which meant detailing a staff radiologist to interpret films on the spot for clinicians, later by opening the film library 24 hours a day.[44] Yet the complaints about slowness of service seemed unremitting. In 1978 a study on improving service in the hospital found that in radiology, "the length of time before reports are received is considered to be unacceptably long; a reduction in patient waiting-time is thought possible."[45] The same theme sounded again in 1983.[46]

What was going on here? Why was the radiology service so irksome to many colleagues? The problem was partly the colleagues' own fault. They insisted on removing films from the department. The radiologists identified "removal of films from the department before radiological interpretation," as a major stumbling block. "Many times these do not return, if at all, till after the patient's discharge. Radiological viewing at that time not infrequently reveals information which would have altered the patient's treatment, had it been recognized." Retaining the films in the department became an ongoing battle in the years ahead.[47]

In 1983 the department tried to figure out the root causes of the continual tardiness in reporting. An audit showed there was a five- to ten-day delay between dictating a report and signing it. The reasons for the delay were all trivial: the computer was often down. Also: "An important factor was the amount of re-typing requested."[48] Yet like the proverbial wanting nail that led to the loss of the kingdom, these small details could result in serious impairments in patient care. Lansdown took steps to bring the reporting time down to forty-eight hours.

How about the urgency with which bad news is communicated to the referring physician? In the old days there was little. Singleton, when once queried about a woman patient who had a shadow on her chest film, said that "the report is placed on the patient's chart and it is expected that the doctor will familiarize himself with it."[49] In fairness to the older generation, there was a good chance these physicians might have seen each other over coffee and discussed the case. Yet in the high-tech medicine of the postmodern hospital, doctors from different services might not meet over coffee. What do we do about positive mammograms? asked one of Lansdown's colleagues. "His concern was the manner in which important reports such as a positive mammogram were delivered to the referring physician.... He thought that these reports should somehow be flagged so as to draw special attention to the significance of the report." At the department staff meeting, "different possible solutions were discussed including red ink, special stamp, and verbal reports."[50]

The devil lies in the details. The enormous growth that radiology experienced after the 1960s compelled the department to overcome multitudes of such micro-problems. As Lansdown stepped down in 1984, the diagnostic side of the department numbered twenty radiologists doing 150,000 examinations a year. That all this had been mastered in a highly professional manner while increasing the department's scientific profile is a tribute to Lansdown's quiet style of administrative competence.

In 1989 Chia-Sing Ho became chief of radiology at the Toronto General Hospital. In 1991 the departments at the General and the Western merged, and from that point Ho was chief of what in 1995—the centennial year—became the Department of Medical Imaging of The Toronto Hospital.

Hospital for Sick Children

The postwar era in radiology at the Hospital for Sick Children began in 1946 with the appointment of John Munn, then thirty-three. Munn was born in 1913 in Ripley, Ontario, and went to medical school at the University of Western Ontario where he graduated in 1938 as a member of the Osler Society, meaning among the top four members of the class. He interned at Hamilton General Hospital, and was then briefly a general practitioner in Northern Ontario. Between 1941 and 1943 Munn did a radiology residency at Toronto General Hospital. After three years overseas with the Royal Canadian Army Medical Corps, he returned with the rank of major to direct the radiology service of the Discharge Centre at Exhibition Grounds in Toronto, processing over a thousand servicemen and -women a day. From there it was an easy step to HSC, where in June 1946 he became assistant radiologist under Rolph. Knowing nothing at this point about pediatric radiology, Munn went down to the Children's Hospital in Boston where he studied for three months with Edward Neuhauser, thence to New York for another stint with pediatric radiologist John Caffey. These were the two big names in pediatric radiology in the States. "I was green as hell as far as pediatric radiology was concerned," said Munn later. "I learned it from books, from Neuhauser and Caffey. Caffey's book on it was very elementary but good." In January 1947 Munn became head of pediatric radiology in Toronto.

Munn turned a new page at HSC. At once he put an end to staff removing films from the department before he had a chance to report them. "I laid down the rule shortly after I got there that either I reported all the material taken or I would resign."[51] There were always fights over this, he said later. He started keeping the films in the department and laid down the law to the tough HSC surgeons.[52] "Robert Wansbrough was bad and liked to pick trouble with the x-ray department. I said to him, all you fellows do is bitch. I don't think anybody had ever talked to him before like that. My secretary said there's going to be hell popping. No there wasn't. Next day he was nice. I was a farmer, tough to get along with. I didn't let myself be intimidated."[53]

Munn put an end to Rolph's practice of irradiating the supposedly enlarged thymus. Beginning around 1924 Rolph had been treating cases of "thymic enlargement," irradiating several hundred every year, apparently on the grounds that an enlarged thymus was causing stridor in babies by compressing the trachea. Once Munn demonstrated to the staff that the thymus normally changed size and shape in the course of respiration, they agreed that the practice should be stopped.[54]

At HSC Munn innovated in several ways. Even before Munn's arrival, the surgeon John Keith had been working on cardiac catheterization. In 1948 Munn, Keith and a technician developed an angiography camera, called the "diagnostic x-ray camera," that could take films at four frames per second to determine whether infants with cyanotic heart disease ("blue babies") were operable.[55] Munn helped inaugurate the hospital's historic interest in fibrocystic disease of the pancreas, making the point he had learned in Boston, that it could be diagnosed radiologically. As Munn later recalled, "They used to say you cannot make a pathological diagnosis from x-ray film. [To make their own diagnosis] the clinicians would pass a tube down the child's esophagus and take a sample of the gastric juices to see if he had duodenal enzymes, the right number, the right kind. That was the way you proved diagnosis they said. You'd hear on rounds that you couldn't do this, couldn't do that. I used to step over the boundaries and set them back."[56] Munn is also remembered, along with John Darte, for fighting against the x-ray machines once set up in shoe stores to check if the shoes were too tight. From 1964 on he joined the ranks of the first radiologic whistle-blowers on child-abuse, establishing radiologic criteria in the "battered child syndrome."[57] To reduce

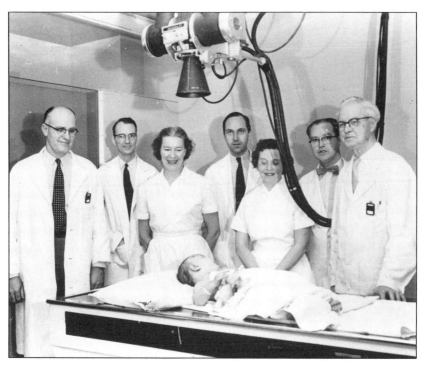

Figure 22. 500,000th x-ray at the Hospital for Sick Children, 1960. Left to right: Dr. John D. Munn (radiologist-in-chief), Dr. Alaric Humphry, Mrs. Phyliss Deakin, Dr. C.A.F. Moes, Mrs. Jean Forward, and veteran technicians Mr. Hugh Menagh and Mr. Les Cartwright. *Hospital for Sick Children Archives.*

cross-infection, he separated the x-ray services for in- and out-patients.[58]

Although not universally admired for his crusty style, Munn was a strong leader. The board of trustees never refused any of his requests. By the time he left the hospital in 1967, he had brought in more powerful equipment that shortened exposure time while better controlling the x-ray beam. He had obtained for the hospital an "X-Omat" that stepped up developing film from one hour to seven minutes. And he equipped the department with image intensification, inaugurating modern fluoroscopy at HSC as Holmes had at the General. At the time of his departure the department consisted of four members, one of whom was Bernard Reilly.

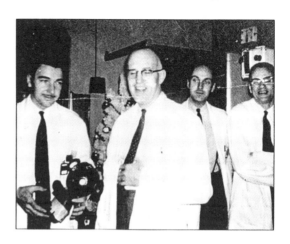

Figure 23.
Bernard J. (Barney) Reilly, radiologist-in-chief, former chief John Munn, Fred Moes and A. Humphry, Hospital for Sick Children, 1968.

In October 1967 Barney Reilly became head of radiology, inaugurating what is even now looked back on fondly as "the Reilly era." This amiable, soft-spoken Scotsman was born in 1926 in Glasgow and earned an MB there in 1949. The following year the Saskatchewan Antituberculosis League brought him to Canada, where he worked first as a sanitarium doctor, then as a GP in Saskatchewan. In the 1950s the demand for radiology was expanding rapidly and the big group-radiology practice in Saskatoon wanted to recruit him as a member. "You had to be a specialist in something," Reilly said later. "General practice as we knew it then was going nowhere." Reilly did a year in pathology at the University of Saskatchewan, then rotated among the city's various hospitals, finally spending a year at Boston City Hospital under Neuhauser as Munn had a decade previously. "Neuhauser was something of a Canadophile," said Reilly (who was Neuhauser's chief resident). In 1959 Reilly returned to Saskatoon to join the group, but pediatric radiology in Saskatoon then was only a blur on the horizon. So Reilly wrote to Munn and got a post at HSC, taking a huge cut in salary. "My salary was less than I'd paid in income tax the year before," he said.

Thus in 1961 Reilly came to the Hospital for Sick Children. The post of chief radiologist had just opened up at the North York General Hospital, then in construction. Reilly tried for it, won the appointment, and took a year off to retool as a general radiologist under Holmes at TGH. In the meantime Munn had stepped down, and Reilly returned to HSC as chief radiologist in 1967.

It was a time of great challenges. HSC's wing on Elm Street was just under construction (finished in 1971), and Reilly had to design a new and much enlarged department. He set out to recruit bright young people, hiring Derek Harwood-Nash, then a resident at TGH and future star neuroradiologist. Reilly brought David Gilday on board, who would establish nuclear medicine at HSC. Under Reilly the department expanded to thirteen radiologists by the late 1970s. "I recruited young people and gave them their head," he later said. "Tell me what you want and I'll get it for you. The trustees accused me of being in the wrong profession. They said I should have been a salesman."[59]

In expanding the department from four to thirteen, Reilly created divisions for pediatric neuroradiology, cardiology, nuclear medicine, gastrointestinal, and genitourinary. He brought in CT scanning. He had said at the outset that ten years as head would suffice. By the time he stepped down in 1978, he had, as colleague Frederic Moes said, "put the place on the map."

Among the subspecialties that thrived under Reilly, one of the most formidable was pediatric neuroradiology. In the late 1930s air encephalography commenced at HSC.[60] By 1948 the hospital was doing over a hundred encephalograms a year and several dozen ventriculograms.[61] Yet the first neuroradiologist as such would come only in 1961, when Evert Kruyff commenced a fellowship year, then stayed on for several years doing research with Munn on tumors in the posterior fossa.[62] (Kruyff, like his fellow neuroradiologist at the Toronto Western Hospital Karel TerBrugge, came from the Netherlands, with a 1947 MD from Amsterdam.)

Yet HSC's neuroradiologist of renown—of such renown that the hospital would signal the publication of his textbook on pediatric neuroradiology as one of the landmark events of the 1970s—was Derek Harwood-Nash. Harwood-Nash was born in 1936 in Bulawayo, Rhodesia, and went to Cape Town for his university career. Captain of the swimming team, sports editor of the "Varsity

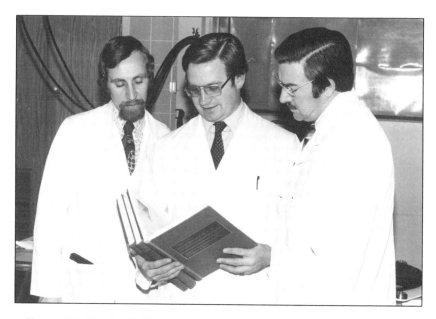

Figure 24. Charles R. Fitz, Derek Harwood-Nash, and Barney Reilly examine a copy of Harwood-Nash's landmark text *Neuroradiology in Infants and Children*, 1976.

Magazine," Harwood-Nash graduated MB in 1960. After an internship year at Cape Town, he came to Toronto in 1962 first as a "fellow," then as assistant resident in neurosurgery under Thomas Morley. Next, Harwood-Nash spent a year as a resident in orthopedic surgery at Sunnybrook. Only in July 1964 did he settle on radiology, and for the next three years trained with Holmes at the General. In 1968 Harwood-Nash became the neuroradiologist at the Hospital for Sick Children, remaining there subsequently. It was at HSC that, aided by Charles R. Fitz, Harwood-Nash did the research for his three-volume textbook in pediatric neuroradiology, published in 1976, which counts as one of the landmark events in the development of the field.[63] In 1978 he became radiologist-in-chief of the hospital. Harwood-Nash went on to become in 1987 president of the American Society of Neuroradiology, and in 1995 received the Gold Medal of the Society for Pediatric Radiology. This represents a lifetime of major achievement and Derek Harwood-Nash became one of the most acclaimed figures in the university department of radiology.

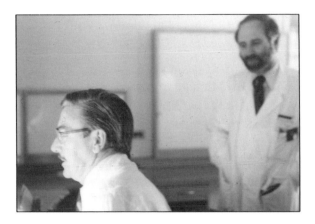

Figure 25.
Barney Reilly and David J. Martin, 1983. Martin established the Ultrasound unit at HSC in 1978.

It is interesting that Alan Daneman, who became radiologist-in-chief at HSC in 1988, had also gone to medical school in South Africa. During his training at Johannesburg, Daneman won the "Harwood-Nash Award."

By the early 1980s the radiology service at HSC had become known all over the world. A review committee found that, "The group has a well recognized international reputation for clinical and academic work." "This is probably the crown jewel of the [university] department."[64]

St. Michael's Hospital

Radiology at St. Michael's Hospital, an institution founded in 1892 by the Sisters of St. Joseph of Toronto, went back to the earliest days. It had been Edmund King, a physician associated with SMH, who was first in Toronto to use the Roentgen apparatus in 1896 (see p. 1-2). There are scattered references in following years to King x-raying patients, though whether the machine was actually located in the hospital is unclear. One source puts the arrival of the x-ray in 1901.[65] In 1902 one of the sisters wrote, "Visited Saint Michael's Hospital today. Saw practical application of the X-Ray. Another laurel for Catholic Science."[66]

Towards 1910, TGH's technologist Frank Fenner called periodically at St. Mike's with his portable x-ray machine tucked into the back of his car. Apparently this arrangement did not suit, for in

1912 the hospital had a new x-ray machine installed with Fenner as the operator.[67]

Like the Toronto General Hospital and the Hospital for Sick Children in the early days, at St. Michael's Hospital too there were long periods without a staff radiologist. Julian D. Loudon, a young internist at the hospital, was mentioned briefly in the records in 1914 (Loudon later became chief physician at St. Mike's and city coroner). Thereafter a series of sisters' names appear, such as Sister de Pazzi in 1914, Sister Felicitas in 1915 and so forth.

Should the hospital get a radiologist? In 1919 the medical advisory board decided against it. With King chairing the meeting and Loudon present, the board considered "the application of Dr. R. S. E. Murray for the position of Pathologist and Roentgenologist to the Hospital." "The feeling of the meeting was opposed to appointing a medical man for interpreting x-ray plates."[68] (Robert Murray had applied for the job just after graduating from the University of Western Ontario; he would end up as a family doctor in various small towns.)

The medical advisory board soon reversed themselves however. Perhaps it was the inability of the sisters to operate and interpret the fluoroscope the hospital had acquired in 1918. In any event, in May 1921 Harold Tovell became the hospital's first real radiologist. Tovell is one of the grand names in the history of radiology in Toronto. Born in 1887 in Peterborough, Ontario, Tovell came to Toronto as a child. He attended high school at St. Andrew's College, then went on at the University of Toronto and Columbia University, where he graduated in medicine in 1912. After postgraduate work in 1913 in Munich, Tovell returned to Toronto just before the outbreak of war and established with Harry B. Anderson a private radiology practice on Bloor Street. (Anderson was another distinguished old name in Toronto medicine, at one point president of the Ontario Medical Association and member of the board of governors of the University of Toronto.) In 1919 Tovell filled in at the radiology department of the Hospital for Sick Children while Rolph was out of the country.[69] At this time Tovell was also involved in writing and research in radiology.[70] In April

1921 he became staff radiologist at St. Mike's at a salary of $200 per month.[71] Why Tovell left the department in 1925 is unclear. He returned to his private practice on Bloor Street—which he now shared with Elizabeth Stewart[72]—, and continued to consult for many years at St. Mike's and at the Wellesley Hospital until double glaucoma claimed his vision in 1937. He died in 1947. Tovell was the archetype of the gentleman physician whose interests were as cultural as they were medical. He followed closely the Canadian artists of the "Group of Seven" and was associated with the Art Gallery of Toronto and Royal Ontario Museum of Archaeology as well as being a member of the Arts and Letters Club.[73]

Tovell's successor at St. Mike's was cut more in the mold of the businessman-radiologist. The three-decade-long Shannon era in the history of radiology at St. Michael's Hospital was inaugurated by Eugene Shannon as in September 1925 he became head of the department. Shannon was born in Toronto in 1897, the son of a prominent oil dealer. He attended Harbord Collegiate (high school), then entered medicine at U of T in 1915. After graduating from the then five-year program, he did two years of postgraduate work in the Department of Physics and TGH, becoming in 1923 one of the first two graduates of the university's new diploma program in radiology (see pp. 122-125).[74] St. Mike's had thus acquired a scientifically-trained young radiologist.

Under Shannon there was a huge step-up in the number of x-ray patients. In 1918, Sisters Felicitas and Carmela had managed to see only a few over a thousand. In 1926, his first full year in office, Shannon saw five times as many (5568). With the move to spacious new quarters in the "E" wing on Victoria Street in 1927, radiology at St. Mike's expanded to include physiotherapy, meaning Alpine lamps and diathermy machines. By 1930, Shannon's department was seeing almost 8000 patients a year.

For three decades Shannon fought with the hospital over the question of his private practice. Before his appointment at SMH he must have been briefly in private practice, for the board stipulated that it would "buy his X-Ray equipment and have it put up in the back of X-Ray Hall." In his original 1925 contract with the board it was stipulated that he should "have no private patients."[75] When he renewed the following year, he was to get $300 a month plus a fifth of the net profits of the department. Nothing more was said, to be sure, about private patients, but the board spelled out what it understood by "full time": "8 a.m. to 5 p.m. with two hours allowed for lunch," plus being on call "when available."[76] There were numerous disputes over his salary in the years ahead, and so it was perhaps with a sense of injustice that in 1938 he opened a private practice on Bloor Street, seconding to it two employees of the hospital department. Yet he remained apparently full-time at the hospital.[77] In 1955 the hospital indicated its unhappiness that Shannon was spending so much time away from work, and that he was employing other hospital radiologists in his private practice who were supposed "to spend their full day in our radiology department." The board wanted Shannon present in the hospital for a minimum of five hours a day.[78] When later that year he signed his next contract, it was with the stipulation that he not employ SMH radiologists in his private office.[79] One does not know how much Shannon realized from this private office, but his hospital billings alone made him in 1959 the fourth-highest-billing radiologist in the province (after the Singleton group, who were first; Louis Harnick at the Toronto Western Hospital was second; Shannon's student Charles Crang in Sudbury was third).[80] Shannon stepped down as chief in 1963. As he retired from the hospital in 1972, someone wrote in the margin of the minutes of the medical advisory board "litigation."[81] The focus of the Shannon years had thus been misdirected from science, and it was perhaps because of this delay that other teaching hospitals had forged ahead of SMH up to that point.

The parlous state of affairs at St. Mike's finally became a concern to the board of governors of the University of Toronto. Somebody from the Board contacted Singleton and asked him if he couldn't send a radiologist from TGH over to beef things up. Singleton thereupon said to Holmes, "You're the choice."

Said Holmes later, "I had come to Toronto only to be at the General Hospital. I had turned down a job at the Sick Kids. So my answer to Singleton was, the University can push me out but they can't push me around. And that was the end of it. I never heard anything more."[82]

In 1955 Shannon accepted that he needed some help but decided to go for quite junior people.[83] In 1957 three junior radiologists were hired: Joseph Sungaila, a medical graduate of Innsbruck in Austria who was just facing his Royal College exams, and two young brothers Bruce and Grant Bird. Grant had graduated in medicine from Toronto in 1951, Bruce in 1952. Grant would shortly move on from St. Mike's to become chief at the Wellesley in 1971.

Bruce Bird became chief of radiology at St. Mike's in 1963, ending the Shannon years. Just as Barney Reilly strode into Sick Kids with reforming zeal, so did Bruce Bird into SMH. He set out to build the subspecialties across the board. By 1971 the hospital had eight staff radiologists, by 1982 twelve. "A review of the Curriculum Vitae of the staff," wrote Bruce Bird in that year, "reveals 43 publications, 2 chapters and exhibits. Approximately 39 papers of 10 to 20 minutes duration have been given...."[84]

Among the hospital's strongest subspecialties was cardiac. Under Norman Patt, a cardiovascular specialist whom Bird appointed in 1964, SMH organized two cardiac catheterization laboratories and acquired a wide reputation for its work in coronary angiography. The hospital also made a name for itself in mammography, an early service beginning in 1972, the hospital then joining the national breast cancer study in 1984.

Thus within a relatively brief compass of time, radiology at St. Michael's Hospital came to be one of the most important programs in the city. Wrote an inspection team in 1979, "The high spirit and morale in the hospital department is evident. The radiologists are concerned and the residents appreciate their training."[85] (One can imagine what such a team would have written of conditions had it called twenty years earlier.) The story is instructive because it establishes again the importance of strong leadership if progress is to be made. Good science and clinical medicine do not just happen.

Toronto Western Hospital

The Toronto Western Hospital was founded in 1896 by a group of twelve physicians from West Toronto as a private hospital. Three years later it became incorporated as a public hospital in a special act of the provincial legislature. In 1926 the Western merged with the Grace Hospital, which is of interest because it was at the Grace (or Toronto Homeopathic Hospital as it was then called) that x-rays first appeared in Toronto.[86] As for the history of the radiology department at the Toronto Western Hospital as such, the paper trail is rather sparse and we know less than about the other hospitals, even though with its then three hundred beds TWH was an important contender. Radiology apparently arrived there in 1924 with the appointment of young Dr. W. Cecil Kruger. Born in Edmonton, Kruger belonged to a kind of radiology family: His brother George was a radiologist at the Woodstock General Hospital and his brother Herbert an X-ray technician at the International Nickel Hospital in Copper Cliff. Cecil himself had first earned a pharmacy degree in Alberta, then graduated in medicine from the University of Toronto in 1923. He learned radiology during an internship year at the Battle Creek Sanatarium in Michigan.[87] A newspaper story in 1937 refers to the Western's "new radiology department," and makes much of a $20 pair of lead-lined gloves Kruger had purchased.[88] So we may infer that in these early days radiology there was not conducted on a grand scale, even though Kruger did have a university appointment.[89]

Associated with Kruger was another young Toronto graduate—also class of 1923 and also a trainee of the Battle Creek Sanitarium—named Wilbur J. Cryderman. Cryderman began his radiology career in Toronto at the Grace Hospital, where he developed a lively research interest in hiatus hernias and duodenal diverticula, and worked up a new x-ray method of examining them. Cryderman later went over to the Western after it and the Grace were united, and was associated with TWH until his retirement in 1959.[90]

Thus Kruger and Cryderman were the founding generation. Kruger remained on staff at TWH until 1950, when vigorous young

Louis Harnick arrived on scene. Among the generation of wartime physicians trained by Richards who went on to become the leadership figures in Canadian radiology, Louis Harnick was one of the most prominent. Harnick was born in Toronto in 1920, attended Jarvis Collegiate Institute, and graduated from U of T in 1943. For the next three years he was stationed with the military in Halifax, in 1946 helping Munn at the Canadian National Exhibition to decommission the troops in their thousands. Harnick then trained in radiology under Kruger at the Western. He spent a year as an extern in radiology at the Massachusetts General Hospital, and also studied at the Karolinska Institute in Stockholm, returning to the Western in 1949. He became chief of the department in 1951.[91] Holmes, who had got to know Harnick in the second of his own three years at Boston and was Harnick's close friend, later said, "Lou Harnick was a very bright guy, well trained.... He ran an excellent department and was very highly regarded by people in all walks of medicine."[92]

Harnick strode on a stage much bigger than TWH. He was one of the founders of M.D. Management, which ran pension plans for physicians all across Canada. He was at one time president of the Canadian Association of Radiologists and, in the early 1970s president of the Ontario Medical Association. He was also a former president of Beth Tzedec Congregation. Louis Harnick thus cut a major figure. In the early years Harnick was keenly interested in academic research.[93] Yet he lost this interest with time and became increasingly absorbed in his private practice in the medical building on Leonard Avenue just across the street from the Toronto Western Hospital. (He also provided radiology services to community hospitals in Huntsville and Bracebridge as well as to the Hillcrest and Queen Elizabeth hospitals in Toronto.[94]) In 1986, the year after Harnick stepped down as chief of the hospital department, the Primrose Club, a men's club of which Harnick had once been president, named him "Man of the Year." Thus by 1985, when Harnick retired as chief, he had been the dominant figure in radiology at TWH for thirty-five years.

This extraordinarily long stewardship had both positive and negative aspects for the development of radiology at the Toronto Western Hospital. On the positive side, Harnick greatly increased the size of the department, from two in 1950 to ten in 1971, the high point of the service's growth. At that point TWH had the second largest radiology department in the city, with a staff that included some quite distinguished figures such as Douglas McFarlane, who in 1968 founded the training program in mammography. In the early years at least, Harnick was a crackerjack administrator, keen on following up problems such as a "badly leaking fluoroscope" on one occasion, on another the failure to notify the surgeons of significant pre-operative chest findings until an hour or so before the operation.[95] The Toronto Western Hospital became first in the city to acquire an "X-Omat" for processing films.[96]

Yet Harnick's philosophy of radiology was quite different from Holmes's, despite their close friendship. He saw the Toronto Western Hospital as primarily a community hospital and radiology as primarily a service department, not an academic one. Indeed he and his colleagues were uneasy about a closer association with the university department. At one meeting, "Dr. Harnick expressed concern with the growing concept of the hospital becoming a central treatment body, to the exclusion of the community doctor. He considered there should be fifty percent community beds and efforts should be made to attract more general practitioners.... He cautioned against the Hospital becoming overpowered by the U. of T. by the allocation of full-time geographic fellows."[97] During the 1960s, when every academic radiologist in the city was talking about expanding service and developing the subspecialties, Harnick spoke out against expansion at the Western. Committee minutes mention "the firm conviction of Dr. Harnick in the X-ray Department that no important addition to service space will be required."[98]

While Holmes had boosted the importance of the basic sciences in radiology, Harnick thought emphasis should be upon training general practitioners. "He thought to be a good radiologist

you had to know how to look after and deal with patients," said
Doug Sanders. "Holmes's basic philosophy was that in your training you must have knowledge of other fields outside of radiology.... Harnick felt that you learned things from talking with the
patients, and unless you fully understood that and dealt with other
physicians on the same basis, you could never be a success in
radiology."[99]

Harnick's philosophy was in many ways a noble one and
worthy of emulation. Yet it led to a marked uninterest in the
development of subspecialty radiology and in training. "Western
didn't push the idea of subspecialty radiology the way we had at
the General," said Holmes. This failure to push ahead in the field,
combined with a severe economic crunch the hospital underwent
in the 1980s, caused a crisis in which the university department of
radiology almost lost its accreditation. At a trustees meeting of the
Toronto General Hospital in 1987, H. V. Stoughton, president of
the hospital, reported "that the Radiology Department at University of Toronto was granted provisional accreditation due to perceived problems of lack of equipment and space at Toronto
Western Hospital. Radiology had been identified as the first priority for support in the implementation of the master plan by the
MAC [medical advisory committee] at the Western."[100] The crisis
was worked through in a number of ways: by letting the dynamic
young Karel TerBrugge come to the fore, by donation from the
private sector of new imaging technology, and, ultimately, by the
merger in 1990 of the Toronto Western Hospital with the Toronto
General Hospital to form "The Toronto Hospital."

In retrospect, Lou Harnick was a complex and controversial
figure. The paper trail leaves a rather harsh picture of him. Yet
people's lives consist of more than paper, and in the recollections
of colleagues Harnick was a man who made a considerable contri-
bution to radiology and to the Toronto Western Hospital. Cardiolo-
gist Susan Lenkei pointed out, for example, that in 1980 Harnick
encouraged the hospital to get the first biplane angiographic unit
in all of Canada. "We had the first totally up to date cardiac
catheterization lab," she said. "He was a very progressive leader,"

she said, "but he didn't want the university to run the hospital."[101]
It is a final positive comment on Lou Harnick's leadership that he
helped initiate the neurointerventional program at the Western,
realizing early in the game that Toronto required this subspecialty,
and that the Western offered an ideal home for it[102] (see p. 165).
These contributions must be weighed in the balance.

Yet in other ways Harnick did not stand out as a leader. And
the reality is that his preoccupation with his private practice, to the
neglect of the hospital department, helped precipitate a major
institutional crisis in one of the city's principal teaching hospitals.
When Harnick stepped down in the summer of 1984, Nabil
Beschai briefly became chief of the department, then Gordon Potts
himself assumed the chiefship at the Western with his arrival in
1985 in Toronto.

The Wellesley Hospital

The Wellesley Hospital was founded in 1911 by Dr. Herbert A.
Bruce, then a distinguished surgeon and later Lieutenant-Governor
of the province. He bought an old mansion at the corner of
Wellesley Street and Homewood Avenue and opened it in 1912 as
his private seventy-two-bed hospital, catering to the carriage trade
of Toronto's wealthy Rosedale district.[103] When visiting Toronto
in 1914 the English surgeon W. Arbuthnot Lane remarked after
seeing the Wellesley, "I don't think we have anything in London
quite like this. We have magnificent hospitals and abundant facilities for treating the unfortunate poor, but we have no place so well
equipped for the unfortunate rich—or should one say the unfortunate well-to-do."[104] Yet as a private hospital, in the early days the
Wellesley was regarded a bit askance by the city's medical establishment. As the board noted in 1916, "The impression among
medical men is that Wellesley Hospital is a private commercial
venture of Dr. Bruce and for this reason [there is] a certain
discrimination against the institution."[105]

Consequently radiology at the Wellesley did not flourish any
more than did the rest of the institution. In 1918 Charles E. Treble,

a U of T graduate of 1901, established an x-ray department in the hospital.[106] He died the following year. Who, if anyone, filled in is unknown, but sometime after 1925 Harold Tovell became the hospital's next radiologist. A long period of stability then began around 1936 with Keith Bonner. A U of T graduate of the class of 1934, Bonner spent two years of postgraduate study in radiology in New York, then came to a post at the Wellesley. He owned his own equipment, for which TGH paid him $25,000 as it took over the Wellesley in 1948.[107] (The Wellesley had in the meantime become a public hospital in 1942.) From 1948 until the hospital again became independent in 1960, its radiology department was part of TGH's, and Kenneth MacEwen, who succeeded Bonner in 1950, was the division chief.

Ken MacEwen, as noted above, had come from the General. After graduating from U of T in 1939, he had spent part of his clerkship and internship years at the Western under Kruger, rotating through the radiology service and serving also as night technician between 1939 and 1941. Once in the RCAF, MacEwen took the radiology cram course at the General, did his military service, then returned to TGH as a staffer. After TGH took over the Wellesley, MacEwen became head of the division, remaining until his retirement in 1971.[108]

Before MacEwen, radiology at the Wellesley was basically a one-man department. Then in the 1960s the hospital expanded to over 600 beds, and by 1967 the radiology department had grown to six staffers, working in six rooms and doing studies on a hundred patients a day. Much of the new imaging equipment—including an image intensifier acquired in 1964— had been donated by the Atkinson Foundation.

The man who succeeded MacEwen in these years of growth was Grant Bird. Grant was born in 1927—a year before his brother Bruce—and grew up in Oshawa, Ontario, in a medical family. He graduated from the University of Toronto in 1951, interned as a resident at several of the Toronto hospitals, as well as fellowing in radiology at the Mayo Clinic between 1954 and 1956. (Bruce fellowed there as well.) Just after his Royal College certification in diagnostic radiology in 1957, Grant Bird spent a year at St. Michael's Hospital, then in 1959 became a staff radiologist at the Wellesley Hospital, where he remained until his retirement in 1990. Between 1971 and 1986 Bird was chief of radiology. Therewith both of Toronto's large east-end hospital radiology departments were simultaneously run by the Bird brothers.

Although the department formally inaugurated a postgraduate training program in 1960, it had few residents (in 1983 none). In terms of scientific accomplishment, between 1976 and 1992 Robin Grey helped give radiology at the Wellesley something of a national profile in angiography and interventional radiology.

Women's College Hospital

The Women's College Hospital occupies something of a special place in the story. The hospital began in 1896 as a small dispensary in Mission Hall at the corner of St. David and Sackville Streets in connection with the Ontario Medical College for Women. In 1910 the dispensary moved to another site on Seaton Street in Toronto's east end, admitting in that year the first patient. By 1911 the hospital had increased to seven beds and three years later the by now twenty-five bed hospital removed to Rusholme Road in Toronto's west end. In 1935 it reached its permanent location as a 250-bed institution on Grenville Street near the city's hospital row.[109] Women's College, as the name suggests, was in the early years for female patients and until the 1960s was staffed entirely by women.

In 1919 Elizabeth Stewart established an x-ray department at WCH. Born in Sandford, Ontario, in 1880, she was the daughter of a Methodist clergyman.[110] She attended high school in North Bay, then graduated in medicine from U of T in 1911, a member of the university's second co-educational class in medicine. She interned at Women's Hospital in Philadelphia, then returned to Toronto to join the medical staff of WCH on Seaton Street and to run a private practice with another female physician. At this point she decided to study radiology, possibly because all the other

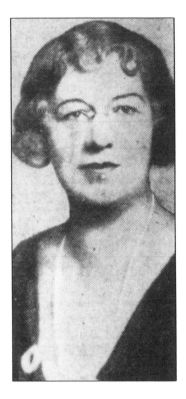

Figure 26.
Dr. Elizabeth Stewart.
Founder of the Radiology
Department at Women's
College Hospital and its chief
radiologist until 1955.
Photograph from the Toronto
Daily Mail and Empire, 5 April
1935

hospitals in the city were acquiring departments and she wanted to keep Women's College abreast of the times. So she spent the years 1918-19 doing radiologic work at the Lennox Hill Hospital in New York and the Johns Hopkins in Baltimore, coming back to Toronto to establish a department of radiology and physiotherapy at WCH at a salary of $664 a year.[111] The hospital board asked the medical advisory committee to organize the radiology service in the form of a committee, with surgeon Jessie Gray as "chairman." Therewith Elizabeth Stewart, "the newly appointed Roentgen Radiographer," became Canada's first female career radiologist (as opposed to Lillias Cringan's brief trajectory at the Hospital for Sick Children, see p. 25).[112] At Women's College, physiotherapy later became added to radiology and Stewart supervised both functions.

Stewart was described in 1941 as being "of jolly appearance, with bright blue eyes and graying brown curly hair."[113] Yet she had suffered the radiation burns characteristic of early radiology and at some point earlier in her life was said to have lost all her hair and to wear a wig.[114] So we may infer that by 1941 (when she became became appointed to the medical board of the Women's Auxiliary Air Force) the hospital's radiology equipment was better shielded. WCH did only diagnostic work; patients in need of therapy were sent to the Dunlap Building of Toronto General Hospital.

Simultaneously with her staff post at WCH, Stewart maintained until 1939 a private practice with Harold Tovell. She served as WCH's radiologist until going on part-time in 1955, though she became by no means inactive in the affairs of the hospital to which she was greatly dedicated. She prided herself on the quality of x-ray work done at the hospital despite "the cramped quarters, the shortage of x-ray rooms, and the constant jiggling made necessary," as one reporter put it.[115]

In 1923 Stewart was joined by Helen Bell-Milburn, who was to become the hospital's breast specialist and chief of the outpatient department. Milburn was born in 1892 in London, Ontario, earned a physics degree at U of T's University College, then graduated in medicine in 1919. Like Stewart, she studied radiology at New York's Bellevue Hospital, and then worked in radiation therapy at TGH between January 1922 and April 1923 (which would make her and not Vera Peters the first female student of Gordon Richards). Milburn came on staff at Women's College in 1923, retiring at the same time as Stewart in 1955.[116] She had married Clement Milburn and called herself by that name.[117]

WCH's first set of radiology equipment was a gift from William Davies, the founder of a prosperous pork-packing firm. Davies had a history of philanthropy to hospitals and women's higher education. Although this donation made for a promising beginning, for decades to come the hospital would be plagued with the financing of new equipment. In 1947 it organized the first major upgrading of its equipment in decades, then another in 1955 as the department moved into new quarters on the second floor of south wing. By this time the pallette of services included two gastric rooms, two general rooms, and a room for cystoscopy.[118]

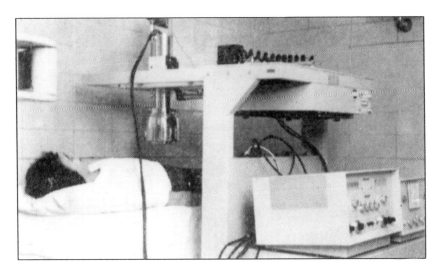

Figure 27. New Isotope equipment at Women's College Hospital, 1962. WCH, *Annual Report, 1962.*

In 1951 physiotherapy had been hived off as a separate department.[119]

With this changing of facilities came a changing of the guard. The two founding mothers stepped down and Elizabeth Forbes became the head of radiology. Born in 1917 in Blenheim, Ontario, after high school in Blenheim, she attended a nearby business school (where in 1935 she won a gold medal in accountancy), then decided to go into medicine. In 1942 she graduated MD from the University of Western Ontario. For the next decade she was a family doctor in London. Like other female radiologists, she turned towards the U.S. for her graduate training in radiology, interning as a resident at Strong Memorial Hospital in Rochester in 1953-54, then coming on staff as the new chief at WCH in 1955. In that year she obtained the Royal College certification in in diagnostic radiology.[120] Under Forbes, in 1969 the radiology department at WCH became a division of the university department of radiology,[121] though in fact it would do little teaching of either graduates or undergraduates. (In 1960 WCH began taking on residents one at a time from the Toronto Western Hospital for 3-month rotations.[122])

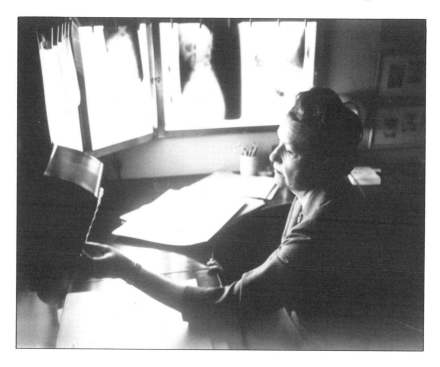

Figure 28. M. Elizabeth Forbes, chief radiologist at Women's College Hospital, 1956-75. WCH was the first hospital in Canada to perform routine mammographic screening, 1963. *Women's College Hospital Archives.*

Forbes brought mammography to Toronto, and routine mammography screening programs to Canada. To place her work in perspective, one recalls that in 1945 Helen Milburn—in collaboration with the British Columbia Cancer Institute in Vancouver—had initiated a screening program for breast cancer. It began as a research project. Milburn and other staff members wanted to determine what relationship existed between physiological changes in the normal breast and the development of breast cancer. They examined a group of volunteer nurses, then followed them for three years. In 1949 the project was widened to volunteers among teachers in the Toronto schools, again, intending to follow a total group of 1600. In the context of this burgeoning involvement in cancer screening, Milburn and Florence McConney established in 1948 a "well women's clinic," examining all comers, half

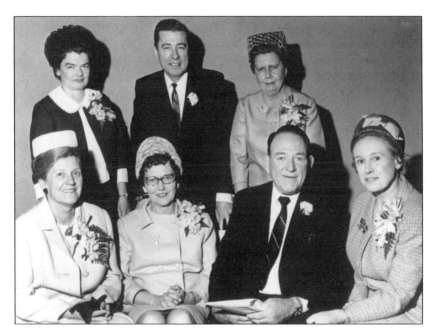

Figure 29. CBC television personality Fred Davis and cancer survivor/spokesperson William Gargan with five cancer specialists from Women's College Hospital at a Canadian Cancer Society fund-raiser, Eaton's College Street auditorium, Toronto, 15 April 1966. Seated left to right: Alice Gray, Vera Peters, Bill Gargan, and Henrietta Banting. Standing, left to right: Ruth Allison, Fred Davis, and Marjorie Davis. *Women's College Hospital Archives.*

the cost of which would be paid by the patient, half by the Ontario Cancer Research and Treatment Foundation. This "well women's clinic" was formally baptized the Cancer Detection Clinic."[123] By 1955, over 16,000 women had been screened, 127 lesions diagnosed.[124] In 1958 McConney stepped down as director and was replaced by Henrietta Banting.[125]

Thus by the time Forbes arrived in 1955 a breast-screening program was already flourishing at Women's College (after 1958 under the direction of Henrietta Banting, who had graduated medicine in 1945, four years after the death of her husband Sir Frederick Banting). What Forbes contributed was instituting in 1963 the first mammography program in Ontario. By 1968 she and Banting were able to publish a review article of the first 1500 cases, somewhat more than half referred from the Cancer Detection Clinic, the others from private physicians.[126] Forbes retired as chief of radiology in 1975. After Henrietta Banting died the following year the hospital's breast cancer centre, now with its own dedicated quarters on the third floor, was named in her honor as the "Henrietta Banting Breast Centre." Eve Fishell became the department's mammographer.[127]

Although the case load had been growing steadily in radiology at Women's College—from 173 patients in 1922 to over 50,000 exams in 1978-79—unfortunately the resources had not.[128] The severely underfunded hospital had not been able to keep pace alongside the Toronto General Hospital. In particular, WCH had no CT scanner and could not afford to upgrade angiography.[129] A crisis arose from the perception that WCH generally was behind the times, and it looked as though Women's College would merge with the General. After much protest (and a new Board), merger was averted. The department received new funding to let it concentrate in the high-risk perinatal area and in mammography. By 1992-93 the department, chaired by Eve Fishell, had a staff of eight (as opposed to two in 1971), a large complement of ultrasound units on site and at the Women's Health Centre, and three mammography units.[130] Amongst the proliferation of Toronto's teaching hospitals, only at Women's College had radiology been able to maintain itself through the strategy of specialization, yet it turned out to be an effective strategy.

Mount Sinai Hospital

The experience of some of the other hospitals might suggest that the appointment of very long-serving chiefs is a bad idea. That conclusion would not be justified for the Mount Sinai Hospital, where an extremely long-serving chief, the resolute Bernard Shapiro, built the department from the two half-time radiologists who were around in December 1955 when he became chief, to one of Canada's largest and most forward-looking departments in 1980 when he stepped down.

The story of Mt. Sinai Hospital goes back to 1923 when a women's charitable group, the Ezra Noshim Society, founded a Jewish community hospital on Yorkville Avenue. It had only thirty-three beds. Records of the earliest days of radiology have been lost, but by the late 1920s or early 1930s David Eisen, who shared a private radiology practice with Cyril Rotenberg on College Street, was reading films half days, sharing the other half with various colleagues.

While many Toronto radiologists had been born in such exotic climes as England and Wales, none before David Eisen had come from Eastern Europe. Born in 1901 in Galicia, a poorish province of the then Austro-Hungarian Empire, Eisen came to Toronto with his family in 1903. He attended Harbord Collegiate, then was admitted to medicine at U of T, graduating in 1922. It is characteristic of the anti-Semitism prevailing in medical circles in Toronto then, that Eisen interned not in the city but at the Hamot Hospital in Erie, Pennsylvania, a Jewish hospital. He then trained further at the Montefiore Hospital in New York City. He returned to Toronto in 1926, first to practice surgery at the Mt. Sinai Hospital, then radiology after the hospital expanded in 1934 and established a department of radiology. Yet Eisen remained essentially a community radiologist. He never received a university affiliation or became involved in research though he must have had scientific ambitions for he earned an MSc at the University of Pennsylvania in 1933. If this surmise about anti-Semitism deflecting his trajectory is correct, one sees what a tragic waste Toronto's earlier pattern of hostility to Jews represented, for thirty years later a man with this profile would almost certainly have had a distinguished scientific career. (In fact that restless energy did find something of an outlet, for he created and kept the archives at Holy Blossom Temple and published his diary as a medical student.[131])

In 1953 the old Yorkville Avenue community hospital gave way to a big new teaching hospital with 330 beds on University Avenue, named the New Mount Sinai Hospital. In view of gaining university accreditation as quickly as possible, the board of directors sought scientific leaders for all the clinical departments, and did so for radiology as well. In 1955 Bernard Shapiro was appointed as the hospital's first full-time radiologist. Shapiro was in every sense an outsider, a Montrealer who had graduated from McGill in 1942 and had interned at the Jewish General Hospital. He went on to train there in medicine and radiology, staying until 1951 as a staffer in order to set up a thyroid uptake laboratory in the radiology department. Then Shapiro moved to Ontario. From 1951 to 1955 he was chief of radiology at the Westminster Hospital in London, Ontario. It was at this time that Sidney Liswood, the administrator of the New Mt. Sinai, began to cast about for a radiology chief for Toronto. Liswood phoned Harnick (as Shapiro later tells the story): "Do you know anybody who would come here?"

Harnick said, "There's a guy Shapiro. I don't know him. You could try."

So Shapiro got a call from Harnick: "They would like to see you at Sinai. Will you come down?"

Shapiro said, "I don't know. I like London, Ontario. It's a nice town."

Harnick said, "Don't be a schmuck."[132]

In 1955 Shapiro took up his new post in Toronto. Eisen became a "consultant." Shapiro found a brand-new department in chaos. "There was no continuity of work," he told the board of directors, "as one man was here during the morning and another in the afternoon. Nor could there be any true loyalty as when one started a case, the other could not follow it to its completion." The hospital planners had lavished large amounts of time on the department's layout and got it all wrong, putting the two cystoscopy rooms right in the central area where radiologists like to have viewboxes and consult with colleagues. Some of the rooms were out of the department entirely, and an expensive head unit that could also serve for pneumoencephalography and cerebral arteriography was so far away that it was seldom used.[133]

In addition to a sense of order, Shapiro also brought to the Sinai a deeply humane philosophy of patient care. "The first thing that

I did when I arrived at New Mount Sinai was to have a meeting with the X-Ray staff. At this time I informed them that I wished all patients to receive courteous treatment. Never under any circumstances was the patient to be chastised or given rough treatment. I told them that they should always remember that people who come to us are ill; they require kindness and consideration." But this news did not go over well with the staff. "I could see they resented being told what to do. They apparently were in the habit of running the department as they pleased. The very next day I overheard the receptionist being extremely rude to a patient on the telephone. She was relieved of her duties and given her week's notice." It is clear then that Shapiro did more than bring academic radiology to what had been a community hospital. He refashioned its corporate culture according to his own understanding of humane medicine—and retained moreover this devotion to patients' well-being throughout his career, at one point lecturing a graduating class of technologists on the importance of treating patients like "human beings and not like pieces of machinery."[134]

Shapiro said that he had never experienced overt anti-Semitism in Toronto. But he, the Montrealer, did find it necessary to become a "Torontonian." As part of preparing for his fellowship exam in the Royal College, in 1957 he took an internal medicine course at the General, then spent two years as a part-time postgraduate fellow in Singleton's service. By the time he took the exam in 1960, he said, "I was Singleton's boy." "When I got the fellowship it said U of T after it and not McGill. I was legally adopted by Toronto."

The volume of work at the Sinai grew very rapidly. In 1956 Shapiro hired Imre Simor, who had graduated in medicine from Munich in 1950 and trained in radiology in London, Ontario. In 1962 Marvin Steinhardt, a Berne MD who had trained at the Western, joined this very international department. In 1970 Murray Miskin arrived, whom Shapiro dragooned for the then unpromising field of ultrasonography. In 1974 Shapiro hired Richard Holgate, the department's first neuroradiologist.

By this time the department was bulging at the seams, as was the whole hospital. Planning for a new hospital began in 1969, and five years later in 1974 the New Mount Sinai Hospital moved a few yards north on University Avenue to become the Mount Sinai Hospital. The radiology department's floor space increased from 5200 to 21,000 square feet.

To facilitate this rapid expansion, the form of remuneration changed in 1966 from salary to fee-for-service, the fees shared from a common pool. In this arrangement lay the seeds of divisiveness, for several members of the department had outside practices, the fees from which did not go into the pool. In 1980 the board of directors forbade radiologists to have outside practices, bringing to a head a serious internal dispute within the radiology department.[135] It was time, in any event, for Shapiro to step down after fifteen years as chief. But before a new chief was willing to take the post, this dispute had to be resolved. It ended in 1981 with the resignation of several valued colleagues.[136] At that point George Wortzman felt able to take the post as the Sinai's next chief of radiology.

But it wasn't just because the department resolved this internal dispute that Wortzman agreed in 1981 to come. It was also because the department acquired a CT scanner. Wortzman, who had come to TGH in 1959, was by this time a distinguished neuroradiologist with a major international reputation (see p. 73 for his career). When in 1981 he accepted the post at the Sinai, it was with the thought "that it would be an easier job as chief."[137] In this, he was to be disappointed.

By the time Wortzman took command, the division of diagnostic radiology had grown to nine full-time radiologists and five specialists in the division of nuclear medicine. The department was doing 115,000 exams a year and had developed a strong program in nuclear medicine and ultrasound (see ch. 5).

The story of the Mount Sinai Hospital is a particularly encouraging one because it demonstrates the importance of leadership. Shapiro with his jocular earthy style and the more patrician Wortzman were both highly effective leaders and navigated the department through shoals that might have torn less well led units asunder.

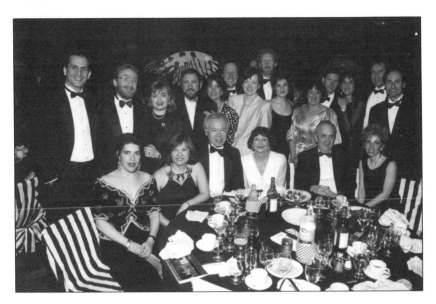

Figure 30. Department of Medical Imaging staff, Mount Sinai Hospital, at the 1995 Brazilian Ball Carnival, Toronto. Standing, left to right: Dr. David Burstein (guest), Dr. Joel and Mrs. Mindy Kirsh, Dr. Shia and Mrs. Jocelyn Salem, Dr. Edward Kassel (radiologist-in-chief), Dr. Lyne Noël de Tilly (guest), Mr. Anthony Sharp, Dr. Karina Bukhanov, Mrs. Jodi and Dr. Murray Asch, Mrs. Kim and Dr. Brian Ginzburg, and Dr. Myles Margolis. Seated left to right: Dr. Eve Cohen, Dr. Roberta and Mr. Nelson Wong, Mrs. Gloria and Dr. George Wortzman, and Mrs. Jodi Margolis. Absent: Drs. Masanori Ichise, Nasir Jaffer, Edward Lansdown, Bernard Shapiro, Imre Simor, and Marvin Steinhardt.

As Edward ("Ted") Kassel became radiologist-in-chief of the Department of Radiological Sciences at MSH in 1993, plans for great expansion lay in the future.

Sunnybrook Hospital

Sunnybrook is the largest of the Toronto teaching hospitals, designed for up to 1600 patients. It is also the only teaching hospital not situated in the downtown core, set rather in a grassy park in a northern suburb. And in the context of the present story it is highly distinctive as well because of its origins. The story goes back to the Christie Street Hospital in downtown Toronto, a veterans' hospital from the time of the First World War. In the passage of time, conditions at the institution had become appalling and in 1942 a committee of Toronto women decided that something must be done, particularly in view of the coming flood of cases from the new conflict. In 1944 it was decided to shift the hospital northward to a farm that had been donated to the city. A new institution would be founded on the site. Sunnybrook Hospital opened officially in 1948, run by the Department of Veterans Affairs. The drama of the Sunnybrook story is how a department that began life mired in the red tape of a department of the federal government became a major teaching center.

When young Desmond Burke (MD Queen's 1932) returned to Canada after four war years as a military radiologist, he wanted to set up in private practice.[138] Unfortunately, in the radiology boom following the war equipment was very scarce and he was unable to locate any, so he accepted a job at the Christie Street Hospital on the condition that he would be allowed to update their anti-quated machines. An extremely energetic figure, Burke was im-mediately successful and, with the caseload of returning veterans, pushed the department to one of the highest volumes in the country. As he was on salary, this was without pecuniary benefit to himself, save that in 1945 the government asked him to design the radiology department of the new Sunnybrook Hospital then under construc-tion. He and his wife built a model of the radiology wing, then "painstakingly made cardboard models of every piece of equip-ment and every desk or chair. They planned doors to open the way they should, laid out entire new designs for darkrooms and therapy chambers." Among the most modern of radiology services in the world, the department opened in 1949 with seven radiologists, fourteen technicians, six stenographers and twelve clinical assis-tants.[139]

Yet things did not go well. The Sunnybrook department had the highest x-ray volume in Canada.[140] But the low salaries paid by the Department of Veterans Affairs made radiologists virtually impossible to retain for any length of time. The Sunnybrook department was a teaching department from the time that it opened.[141] Yet the chaos among the staff meant that interns and residents often went unsupervised and untaught.[142] Consequently it was difficult to get house staff to come up to the lovely, ultra-modern setting, where everybody was run off his feet. Dean Joseph MacFarlane at the Faculty wanted to get John Munn at the Hospital for Sick Children to come up and help out, but Munn refused.[143] Meanwhile, "The interns have had to do a great deal of reporting without the supervision of seniors," lamented one report, which also noted "the loss of four experienced interns and their replacement by totally green trainees...."[144]

In 1957 Burke threw up his hands and became a staff radiologist at a tranquil community hospital. Into this unpromising situation walked the idealistic young Kenneth Hodge. Hodge, born in 1921 at Tunbridge Wells in England, had graduated MB from Guy's Hospital in 1947. He trained in radiology at Guy's Hospital and at the Radcliffe Infirmary in Oxford, receiving his English diploma in 1950. After a year in Dallas, Hodge moved to Canada as a senior resident in radiology at TGH. He had been on staff at the General and Sick Kids for several years when the chiefship at Sunnybrook opened up.[145]

Hodge arrived at Sunnybrook with a vision of organizing a scientific teaching department. For example, in praising colleague Donald Brown to the hospital superintendent, Hodge said, "Dr. Brown is one of those rare people who are prepared to accept an income a little lower than they could obtain elsewhere in order to work in a department such as we envisage at Sunnybrook, and I would, therefore, like to make every effort to attract him here...." Hodge continued, "We are virtually in the process of building this department, and I would like to see good men grow with it."[146] Hodge made an effort to reintegrate the department into the university training program,[147] his predecessor having despaired of accomplishing much in the way of medical education.

Hodge tried hard to upgrade the equipment, for example in 1959 bringing cinefluorography to the hospital (a Toronto first).[148] He toyed with acquiring the first-generation image intensifiers that already in 1957 were on the market (though decided to wait until the screens improved).[149] "Hammers are clattering and electri-

cians' songs and swear words echo through the corridors," he told
a Montreal colleague in 1959. "The machines are lying in their
crates in the bay opposite the [film] museum and instead of
avoiding the eyes of sweating fluoroscopists fuming about the
quality of the films or the latest breakdowns, I just keep a gleaming
new piece of machinery just where they can trip over it when they
stagger swearing out from a particularly juicy barium enema."[150]
Thus he did his best. Unfortunately, Hodge too was overwhelmed
by the problems that had defeated his predecessor, and in 1961 fled
to the Chedoke General Hospital in Hamilton. But Hodge established firmly at Sunnybrook the doctrine that radiology at a teaching hospital should be a full-time proposition, an opportunity for
scientific growth based on the "wealth of excellent clinical material, and first-rate clinicians" that the hospital offered.[151]

A fundamental change in Sunnybrook's situation occurred in
1966 as the University took the hospital over from the federal
government for a payment of one dollar. At this point the constant
"chopping and changing around" which Hodge had deplored came
to an end as the radiologists began earning competitive salaries.
James N. Harvie followed Hodge as chief until 1968, at which
point Donald McRae arrived from Montreal to head the department.

McRae is one of the great names in the history of Canadian
radiology, and was at one time the leading international figure in
the radiology of the base of the skull and the cervical spine. He
was born in Toronto in 1912 and attended Oakwood Collegiate
(high school) before studying medicine at the University of Western Ontario, where he graduated in 1938. McRae then trained in
radiology and, like so many men of his generation, spent the next
four years in the navy. In 1945 he became chief of radiology at the
Montreal Neurological Institute and assistant professor of radiology at McGill. It was at the MNI that he acquired his worldwide
reputation. With the onset of separatist political troubles in the late
1960s, and perhaps motivated by the desire to direct a department
at a big teaching hospital, McRae moved in 1967 from Montreal

to Toronto, becoming chief of radiology at Sunnybrook and professor at the University.

McRae was one of those individuals of whom loving stories are told. He was a quiet and soft-spoken man who cut a most gentlemanly figure. Wortzman recalled him from Montreal days as "a kind of Scottish-Presbyterian type. He said he liked working at the MNI because Wilder Penfield and William Cone both drove Chevies."[152] "If McRae had a weakness at all," said his colleague Harry Shulman, "it was that he didn't fit in with the kind of underhanded backstabbing common in hospitals." McRae would walk about with a magnifying glass that had both a magnifying and minifying lens—so that he could inspect films from up close and from far away. "We used to know when he'd looked at a film," said Shulman, "because there'd be blue-wax crayon marks on it."[153]

Yet actually reading films with McRae could be a bit of an ordeal. "Don was so thorough it was unbelievable," said Wortzman. "He was the most methodical, careful worker. If there was a big stack of films on one patient, he would start at the earliest film ever taken on that patient, then go to the next one and look at it, and on and on till the present study. The next day the patient would have a new study. He would start the bag off again from the very beginning. As a resident it would drive you crazy." Yet behavioral tics or not, McRae became known internationally as an "uncanny diagnostician," in the terms of radiology historian E. R. N. Grigg, who ranked McRae alongside such well-known figures as chest radiologist Benjamin Felson.[154] McRae was a past president of both the Canadian Association of Radiologists and the American Society of Neuroradiology. He retired from Sunnybrook in 1977 and died in 1982 of a heart attack at age seventy.

One of the people McRae had brought from Montreal was John Campbell. Campbell, who stemmed from a medical family in Halifax (his father was once deputy health minister of Nova Scotia), had graduated in 1958 from Dalhousie as gold medalist.[155] He trained at the Victoria General Hospital in Halifax then ended up at the Royal Victoria Hospital in Montreal where he became internationally-known as a specialist in uroradiology. As one of McRae's young stars, he was an obvious candidate to succeed McRae and in 1977 became chief of the now nine-person department. A 1983 review assessed the department as being "very powerful."[156]

With Campbell's untimely death of cancer in 1984 at age fifty-four, Harry Shulman became chief of the department. Shulman, a University of Toronto graduate (1966) who had trained at New York Hospital-Cornell Medical Center, then come on staff at Sunnybrook in 1971, was aware of maintaining a long and distinctive Sunnybrook tradition. "From the beginning," he said in an interview, "all the staff here have been full-time university people. This has generated a greater feeling of commitment. Our reputation for excellence in teaching is due to the fact that our people had no outside office interests."

Of the various leadership patterns in the history of radiology in Toronto—charismatic under Richards, inspiring by example as in the cases of Reilly, Shapiro and Holmes, or anti-leaders such as Shannon—Sunnybrook is an example of leadership by what was essentially good fortune: The hospital got, in the form of people like Hodge, much better leaders than it had any right to expect under the circumstances. Sunnybrook had changed greatly by the time McRae arrived on the scene. Yet nonetheless, it was a piece of good fortune that the political tumult in Montreal in the late '60s made people of McRae's stature think of looking elsewhere. And if McRae had not come to Toronto, Campbell would probably not have come to the city either. The entire story illustrates how difficult it is to plan for success.

Endnotes

[1]Percy Ghent, "Dr. Gordon E. Richards, a Tribute," *Focal Spot,* 6 (Jan., 1949), pp. 16-17, see p. 16.
[2]TGH Board, undated staff list from 1949, p. 1690.
[3]Department of Radiology, University of Toronto, *Annual Report, 1989-1990,* p. 6.
[4]TGH, *Annual Report, 1953,* gives the figure for 1950 as 32,544 examinations, including the Wellesley Hospital.

[5] Arthur S. Singleton, "The Roentgenological Identification of Victims of the 'Noronic' Disaster," *AJR*, 66 (1951), pp. 375-384.

[6] Percy Ghent, "X-Ray Aids Identification of Noronic Victims," *Telegram*, Oct. 4, 1949, p. 6; *Globe and Mail*, Jan. 5, 1950, p. 2.

[7] Malcolm R. Hall, "Arthur Carman Singleton," *Radiology*, 92 (1969), p. 182.

[8] R. Brian Holmes interview, June 3, 1994.

[9] Memorandum within the Ontario Hospital Services Commission from J. B. Neilson to Walter Hardacre, June 26, 1959, p. 6. In the Archives of Ontario, RG 10-221-1-135, box 11.

[10] Holmes interview.

[11] Edward Lansdown interview of May 2, 1994.

[12] TGH MAB, Dec. 22, 1948. After Singleton and Hall had left the meeting, it was revealed that Urquhart had opened the question up.

[13] TGH Trustees, Oct. 4, 1950, p. 1738.

[14] A copy of Singleton's letter is attached to TGH Trustees, Jan. 8, 1952.

[15] TGH Trustees, May 6, 1953.

[16] Holmes and the other juniors asked Singleton if they should resign as well to show solidarity "or just keep our noses down." Holmes interview, Apr. 25, 1994.

[17] Holmes interview, June 3, 1994.

[18] Holmes interview, Apr. 20, 1995.

[19] Department of Radiology, "Presentation to Interdepartmental Planning Co-ordination Committee, Toronto General Hospital," May 25, 1966, p. 32; in files of Department of Diagnostic Imaging, The Toronto Hospital.

[20] University of Toronto, Faculty of Medicine, *Report of the Dean, 1965-1966*, p. 103.

[21] Holmes interview, June 3, 1994.

[22] Personal communication of Holmes to author, Apr. 24, 1995.

[23] TGH staff list for diagnostic radiology for 1967-68 shows, in addition to Holmes, D. E. Sanders, R. F. Colapinto, E. L. Lansdown, R. A. Lobb, R. M. Parrish, G. Wortzman, and B. J. Reilly, plus five voluntary assistants.

[24] TGH Trustees, Jan. 17, 1968, p. 2780; May 8, 1968, p. 2801.

[25] TGH MAB, Aug. 10, 1970.

[26] *Report of the Dean, 1968-69*, p. 156.

[27] TGH Trustees, Oct. 26, 1938.

[28] Douglas Sanders interview of Dec. 28, 1994.

[29] TGH Trustees, Sept. 3, 1969, p. 2895.

[30] Wortzman interview.

[31] Sanders interview.

[32] Sven Ivar Seldinger, "Catheter Replacement of the Needle in Percutaneous Arteriography: A New Technique," *Acta Radiologica*, 39 (1953), pp. 368-376.

[33] *Toronto Star*, Jan. 6, 1961, p. 2.

[34] R. Brian Holmes and D. J. Wright, "Image Orthicon Fluoroscopy of a 12-inch Field and Direct Recording of the Monitor Image," *Radiology*, 79 (1962), pp. 740-751.

[35] TGH Trustees, Nov. 2, 1960, p. 2370.

[36] Sanders interview.

[37]Douglas E. Sanders et al., "Mediastinal and Pulmonary Angiography as an Aid in Determining the Resectability of Primary Lung Cancer," *Canadian Journal of Surgery*, 2 (1959), pp. 147-155; "Angiography as a Means of Determining Resectability of Primary Lung Cancer," *AJR*, 87 (1962), pp. 884-891.

[38]Lansdown interview.

[39]Ronald Colapinto interview of Mar. 2, 1995.

[40]TGH Trustees, June 5, 1963, p. 2528; Jan. 7, 1964, p. 2559.

[41]See for example TGH MAB, Mar. 1, 1973, where surgeon Wilfred Gordon Bigelow requests a third room for coronary angiography.

[42]Wilfred G. Bigelow, *Cold Hearts: The Story of Hypothermia and the Pacemaker in Heart Surgery* (Toronto: McClelland and Stewart, 1984), pp. 131, 202 n. 13.

[43]Richard S. Heilman, "What's Wrong with Radiology," *NEJM*, 306 (1982), pp. 477-479, quote p. 478.

[44]TGH MAB, June 15, 1967; May 15, 1969.

[45]TGH Trustees, Feb. 14, 1978, p. 3797.

[46]TGH MAB, Mar. 3, 1983.

[47]"Presentation to Interdepartmental Committee," 1966, p. 14.

[48]TGH, Department of Radiological Sciences, Minutes, Oct. 27, 1983. File in departmental office.

[49]TGH MAB, Feb. 19, 1953.

[50]Department of Radiological Sciences, Minutes, July 12, 1984.

[51]Munn to Holmes, Dec. 21, 1993. Papers in possession of Munn Family.

[52]For some of Munn's directives see HSC MAB, Jan. 20, 1947, on not removing films before they were reported; Apr. 9, 1947, on storing films in a locked room and on not removing them from the premises without authorization; Oct. 8, 1947, on filling out requisitions properly.

[53]John Munn interview of Oct. 17, 1994.

[54]See HSC *Annual Report, 1924*, p. 38; 1928, p. 56; etc. On the apparent rationale see Munn to Holmes.

[55]See *Globe and Mail*, May 25, 1948, p. 5. John D. Keith and John D. Munn, "Angiocardiography in Infants and Children: New Technic," *Pediatrics*, 6 (1950), pp. 20-32.

[56]Munn interview.

[57]In December 1964 Munn gave a presentation at Osgoode Hall Law School on "Battered Child Syndrome," the first of a series of public appearances on the subject.

[58]Note, [HSC] *Paediatric Patter*, Apr. 1962, p. 2.

[59]Bernard Reilly interview, Mar. 1, 1995.

[60]HSC, *Annual Report, 1938-39*, p. 67. The procedure was evidently recent, though this may not have been the first year.

[61]HSC, *Annual Report, 1948*, p. 69.

[62]Evert Kruyff and John D. Munn, "Posterior Fossa Tumors in Infants and Children," *AJR*, 89 (1963), pp. 951-965.

[63]Derek C. Harwood-Nash, *Neuroradiology in Infants and Children*, 3 vols. (St. Louis: Mosby, 1976).

[64]Undated leaves from the report of a university review committee, included in a binder kept in the Dean's office entitled "Radiology Review, 1983," p. 120.

[65]Irene McDonald, *For the Least of My Brethren: A Centenary History of St Michael's Hospital* (Toronto: Dundurn Press, 1992), p. 115.

[66]"Annals of Sisters of St. Joseph," 1902, vol. 1851-1914, p. 311 (entry for Apr. 2, 1902), SMH Archives.

[67]The basic source for the history of radiology at SMH between 1912 and 1948 is a notebook in the hospital archives, compiled by Sister Rita Mary Smith, box 1031.

[68]SMH MAB, Sept. 8, 1919, p. 93.

[69]HSC MAB, Mar. 24, 1919.

[70]Harold M. Tovell, "The X-Ray in the Diagnosis of Pulmonary Tuberculosis," read at the 19th Annual Convention of the Canadian Association for the Prevention of Tuberculosis, Oct. 9, 1919; copy in Tovell's file in the University of Toronto Archives.

[71]SMH Board of Governors, Apr. 20, 1921.

[72]See Elizabeth L. Stewart and Harold M. Tovell, "Idiopathic Menorrhagia and X-Ray Therapy," *CMAJ*, 13 (1923), pp. 745-748.

[73]Sources on Tovell include an interview with his son, Vincent Tovell, Jan 20, 1994; obituary, *Telegram*, Oct. 16, 1947, p. 3.

[74]Information on Shannon's life from his clipping file in the University of Toronto Archives.

[75]SMH Board of Governors, Nov. 20, 1925.

[76]SMH Board of Governors, May 28, 1926.

[77]See the radiology "Notebook" at SMH, entries for 1938 and after.

[78]SMH MAB Aug. 17, 1955.

[79]SMH MAB, Oct. 3, 1955.

[80]Archives of Ontario, 1959, "Memorandum."

[81]SMH MAB, Jan. 3, 1972.

[82]Holmes interview of Apr. 20, 1995.

[83]SMH MAB, Jan. 7, 1955.

[84]"Five Year Review—St. Michael's Hospital, Department of Diagnostic Imaging, Oct. 5, 1982," p. 6. SMH Archives, X, accession 806.

[85]Department of Radiology, Faculty of Medicine, "Departmental Survey 1979," see SMH entry, p. 4.

[86]See Jesse Edgar Middleton, *The Municipality, of Toronto: A History*, 3 vols. (Toronto: Dominion, 1923), vol. 2, pp. 640-641; Ontario Department of Health, *The Hospitals of Ontario* (Toronto: Ball, 1934), pp. 140-141.

[87]See Kruger's obituary, *Focal Spot*, 11 (1954), p. 223.

[88]"Modern Knight of the Hospital Takes Tip from Knights of Old," *Toronto Star*, Feb. 22, 1937, p. 21.

[89]Sources for Kruger's life include obituaries in the *CMAJ*, 72 (1955), p. 58; *Globe and Mail*, Nov. 11, 1954, p. 8, and his file in the Department of Graduate Records of the University of Toronto Archives. After leaving TWH he became head of radiology at the Humber Memorial Hospital as it was opened in 1950. Kruger died of a heart attack at age 53.

[90]C. W. Harris, "Dr. Wilbur James Cryderman: An Appreciation," *CMAJ*, 95 (Dec. 10, 1966), p. 1271. The obituary gives Cryderman's retirement date as 1964, but the minutes of the TWH MAB meeting of Apr. 14, 1959, say that he will be retiring this year because he has reached the age limit.

[91]For the facts of Harnick's life see obituary, *Toronto Star*, May 17, 1988, p. A21.

[92]Holmes interview.

[93]See University of Toronto, *Report of the Dean, 1951-52*, p. 53.

[94]See the listing of radiology billings for 1959 in Archives of Ontario (RG 10-221-1-135, box 11), as well as a similar list for 1971 (RG 10-221-2-809, box 55. "Radiologists' Contracts...").

[95]TWH MAB, Dec. 10, 1957; Apr. 13, 1954.

[96]"Machine Speeds X-Ray Films," *Globe and Mail*, May 3, 1958, p. 2.

[97]TWH MAB, Aug. 14, 1967.

[98]TWH MAB, Apr 25, 1961, p. 5.

[99]Douglas Sanders interview, Dec. 28, 1994.

[100]TGH Trustees, Jan. 20, 1987, p. 6683.

[101]Susan Lenkei interview, May 5, 1995.

[102]Karel TerBrugge interview of May 6, 1995.

[103]For an upbeat history see Joan Hollobon, *The Lion's Tale: A History of the Wellesley Hospital, 1912-1987* (Toronto: Irwin, 1987), passim.

[104]"Toronto's Most Luxurious Hospital," *Saturday Night*, June 6, 1914, p. 32.

[105]Minute Book, 1911-19, entry of May 28, 1916. In WH Archives.

[106]"Short History of the Wellesley Hospital," c. 1962, p. 1. Manuscript in WH Archives. Treble also ran the radiology service of the Grace Hospital, and while at work in the department there he died of an evident heart attack. *Toronto Star*, Oct. 28, 1919.

[107]TGH Trustees, Dec. 6, 1950.

[108]On MacEwan's life, see G. S. Bird to Dorothy Arnot, Oct. 6, 1977, WH Archives.

[109]For basic facts of WCH's history see WCH, *Annual Report, 1926*, p. 4; see also Martin Kendrick and Krista Slade, *Spirit of Life: The Story of Women's College Hospital* (Toronto: WCH, 1993).

[101]See clippings in Stewart's biographical file at the University of Toronto Archives.

[111]See WCH, *Annual Report, 1920*, pp. 5-6; *Annual Report, 1926*, p. 29.

[112]WCH MAB, Aug. 26, 1919.

[113]"Woman Doctor is Appointed to New Board," *Telegram*, Oct. 7, 1941.

[114]Interview with Vincent Tovell, Jan. 19, 1994.

[115]"Women's College Hospital Plans Five New X-Ray Rooms," *Toronto Star*, Aug. 14, 1932. This account of Stewart's life is based on information in Rose Sheinin and Alan Bakes, *Women and Medicine in Toronto since 1883: A Who's Who* (Toronto: University of Toronto, 1987), p. 95, and on information in her biographical file in the University of Toronto Archives.

[116]Curiously, Milburn seems to have received a formal appointment as "X-Ray associate" only in 1932, "to recognize the unique capacity in which those so recommended have already served." See WCH MAC, Dec. 7, 1932.

[117]Milburn obituary, *Toronto Star*, Sept. 23, 1986, p. A9. Sheinin & Bakes, *Women and Medicine in Toronto*, p. 71.

[118]WCH, *Annual Report, 1955*, p. 5.

[119]"Report of the Department of Radiology for 1951," WCH Archives.

[120]On Forbes's life see Sheinen & Bakes, *Women in Medicine*, p. 28.

[121]WCH MAC, Jan. 7, 1969 Despite Holmes's recommendation, Forbes had second thoughts because she herself did not desire a university appointment (pp. 1, 3).

[122]WCH MAC, May 3, 1960.

[123]OCTRF, *Annual Report, 1949*, pp. 10, 93-94.

[124]OCTRF, *Annual Report, 1955*, p. 34.

[125]WCH, *Annual Report, 1958*. Banting came to the hospital in 1949 or '50. WCH MAC, Apr. 12, 1949, upon Banting's request for a position on the Ob/Gyn staff. "We will be happy to have her on the Staff as soon as she returns from China."

[126]M. Elizabeth Forbes and Henrietta Banting, "An Assessment of Mammography," *JCAR*, 18 (1967), pp. 478-479.

[127]WCH, *Annual Reports, 1975, 1976.*

[128]WCH, *Annual Reports, 1922,* p. 14; *1979,* p. 7.

[129]See "Trauma of a Hospital Merger," *Toronto Star*, Nov. 20, 1989, p. A2. They were promised a CT scanner by 1995.

[130]University of Toronto, Department of Radiology, *Annual Report*, 1992-93, p. 37.

[131]This account of Eisen's life is based on his *Diary of a Medical Student* (Toronto: Canadian Jewish Congress, 1974), pp. 1-4, 99-101; see also his obituary, *Toronto Star*, June 19, 1988, p. A28; also information in scattered medical directories.

[132]Shapiro interview, Jan. 24, 1995.

[133]MSH Directors, Shapiro report of Sept. 30, 1955.

[134]"X-Ray Patients 'Aren't Machines,'" *Toronto Star*, May 18, 1963, p. 69.

[135]MSH Directors, Sept. 30, 1980.

[136]MSH Directors, Mar. 17, 1981.

[137]Wortzman interview, Dec. 14, 1994.

[138]On Burke's life see the obituary in the *Toronto Star*, Apr. 12, 1973, p. 51; and "... New X-Ray Technique," *Telegram*, July 19, 1949, p. 4. Burke was also a noted marksman.

[139]*Telegram,* July 19, 1949.

[140]Burke to C. MacLeod, May 7, 1954. Sunnybrook Health Science Centre Archives.

[141]*Report of the Dean, 1948-49*, p. 43. In 1948 as well, Sunnybrook received Royal College approval for graduate training in diagnostic radiology. RCPS Council, Nov. 25-26, 1948, p. 57.

[142]The correspondence among Kenneth Hodge, the superintendent of the hospital, and the DVA gives considerable insight into these relationships. Preserved in SHSC Archives.

[143]HSC MAB, Dec. 21, 1949.

[144]Desmond Burke to C. MacLeod, June 21, 1957.

[145]See his obituary in *CMAJ*, 108 (1973), p. 359.

[146]Hodge to MacLeod, Oct. 29, 1957, p. 4.

[147]Hodge to Singleton, June 3, 1958.

[148]Hodge to Jean Bouchard, July 23, 1959.

[149]Hodge to Bouchard, Aug. 27, 1957.

[150]Hodge to Bouchard, Apr. 13, 1959.

[151]Hodge to Bouchard, June 24, 1959.

[152]Wortzman interview. Penfield, of course, was the great neurosurgeon, Cone the neurologist.

[153]Harry Shulman interview of April 11, 1995.

[154]E. R. N. Grigg, *The Trail of the Invisible Light* (Springfield: Thomas, 1965), p. 718.

[155]For Campbell's obituaries see *Toronto Star*, Oct. 19, 1984, p. A10; *Globe and Mail*, Oct. 20, 1984, p. 20.

[156]"Radiology Review," 1983, p. 119.

Chapter Four

Training Radiologists

A t the very beginning it was by no means evident that radiology should be a special discipline. At the University of Pennsylvania the training time required to master the discipline was about eight hours. One day in 1902 one of the professors at Penn asked young Henry Pancoast, "How would you like to try the x-ray work?" Pancoast agreed. "In training for the new work, it was necessary to spend eight to ten hours with Dr. Goodspeed, Professor of Physics," Pancoast wrote later. "At the expiration of the time, he told me that was all he knew of the subject and that any further knowledge would have to be gained through experience...."[1] That was the end of Pancoast's training.

In Toronto things were little better. In 1910 the council of the College of Physicians and Surgeons of Ontario was discussing whether the x-ray should be included in the medical curriculum. "No university today is teaching the Roentgen Ray," said Edmund King, who introduced x-rays to Toronto in 1896. "The reason is that the Universities cannot or will not supply the material to teach Roentgen Ray, or they will not or cannot get the men to teach it." Another council member said that every country hospital in Ontario had an x-ray machine. "But who is to teach the medical men in charge of that instrument how to use it.... It is an important factor that the X-Ray should be known to all medical men today. They have to go out of the country to learn it."[2]

Yet Ontario's medical schools did not rise at once to the challenge. They organized no university radiology departments, and hospital x-ray departments continued to be in the hands of technicians. One Canadian observer slaked the hospitals' tendency to avoid hiring radiologists, leaving their x-ray departments to technicians, a practice that let the hospitals save money but rested "on the patently fallacious assumption that every visiting doctor is competent to make his own roentgenological diagnosis."[3]

What created a sense that interpreting the X-ray plates was a legitimate medical speciality—a task of the university medical schools—was the First World War. The army itself trained many young physicians to be radiologists,[4] and they, like Gordon Richards, filtered back from the front to take hospital jobs, and thence to pressure the universities to incorporate radiology in the undergraduate and postgraduate curriculums.

The Diploma Course

In July 1919, at the Faculty of Medicine, a committee of the heads of clinical departments convened. These were the big names of the faculty: Duncan Graham, the chair, who had just become the professor of medicine; Gibb Wishart, the professor of oto-laryngology, and the surgeon Alexander Primrose. "It was determined to recommend that Radiology be made a separate Department of the University in charge of a Lecturer and Demonstrator," the committee decided. Richards was to draw up specifications for the committee.[5] Four months later in November 1919 Richards was appointed "Head of the Department of Radiology in the Faculty of Medicine" with the title of Lecturer (in December he was upgraded to "Associate in Radiology").[6]

In 1920 the Department received its formal organization with Richards as head and Dickson and Rolph classed as "clinicians." Richards would give lectures to the undergraduates, Dickson clinics in gastrointestinal radiology; Rolph at HSC was to offer clinics in pediatric radiology. TGH was supposed to organize a "house service" in radiology with the recommendation "that it be one of the regular rotating services."[7]

Thus radiology became a university department, for the little it was worth. Faculty budgets in the coming years would reflect token allocations for Richards and for a demonstrator as faculty teachers, though in reality the vast bulk of teaching done by department members over the years went unremunerated. With radiology properly constituted as a department, the faculty was able to offer graduate instruction in the form of a diploma course.

In the 1920s voices started to become loud on behalf of formal training for radiologists. "Medical radiology has grown up as an ugly and distorted infant," declared one prestigious radiologist at the Mayo Clinic. "The general level of the specialty is not high, and workers in this field may often be heard to bewail the faint respect with which their efforts are viewed by their fellow physicians in other specialties."[8] What was needed, said the author, was courses comparable to those offered in Europe.

In 1922 the University of Toronto inaugurated a one-month "short course" on radiology offered three times a year, and a diploma training program on the British model, the first of which had been mounted in Cambridge in 1920.[9] Co-operating with J. C. McLennan, the professor of physics, Richards organized a program of instruction for both. The fee for the short course was $100, for the diploma course $400.[10] (After Stanley Ryerson had reported at a meeting of medical educators on the design of Toronto's diploma course, McGill University decided to adopt one too.[11])

The announcement of the short course caused considerable interest among medical practitioners. Wrote one physician from Bay City, Michigan, "Would like to take about one week's special study in X-ray during the first week of October [1922]. Kindly let me know if I can do this at Toronto."

Secretary of the Faculty Stanley Ryerson responded that the course lasted a month, not a week: "The Chairman of the Committee on Graduate Studies states that they could not give a course of one week that would be satisfactory."

The applicant persisted, again omitting the first-person pronoun: "Cannot possibly take all this, can only take one, or at most two weeks.... What I want is how to operate the machine well, read plates and do the more elementary work—no advanced work."

Ryerson ended the exchange by saying that a month was the minimum. "It is for such graduates as yourself that these short courses are planned."[12]

In 1923 the program produced its first two graduates, Eugene Shannon who shortly progressed to St. Michael's Hospital (see p. 89) and Omer Hague, who became Richards' first resident, then returned to his native Winnipeg.[13] For the first time the Faculty of Medicine was involved in training radiologists.

Yet the diploma program ended up training primarily non-academic radiologists. The academic radiologists who came along after World War II mainly aspired to become fellows of the Royal College of Physicians and Surgeons rather than bearers of a university diploma (though many picked up the diploma on their way to the FCRP). Rather, the diploma program trained people to do radiology work at community hospitals.

From the very outset, the radiologic education of the broad masses of physicians had been an issue. Specialty training was seen as something for the offspring of the middle classes, general practice was for poor boys. But poor boys had a right to know how to interpret X-rays too. As the president of the College of Physicians and Surgeons, Eldridge T. Kellam of Niagara Falls, said in 1924, "Not all our students are sons and daughters of wealthy scions, hence it behooves us to see that when they leave our college halls they are competent to take up the work and responsibilities of their profession. The rich man's sons are able to improve their position by hospital work and post-graduate work." Kellam wanted GPs to "be qualified to do their own laboratory work, deprived as they will be of the opportunities of the larger centres. In passing I make bold to mention X-ray training...."[14]

In the area of radiology at least, Kellam got his wish. The graduates of the U of T diploma program came in mainly as family physicians and graduated to become service-oriented radiologists outside the teaching system. "The majority have come from the ranks of general practice and are interested in returning to community practice of radiology," Holmes told the Dean of Medicine in 1966.[15]

The radiology department made some attempt to keep the diploma course abreast of the times, lengthening it to two years in 1949, in combination with internship. To keep pace with trends in England, they changed the name of it in that year from "Diploma of Radiology" to "Diploma of Medical Radiology." This usage was "in keeping with that of the English Colleges and the English Conjoint Board."[16]

By the 1960s the diploma program was turning out five to ten graduates a year. Candidates were based at one of the five teaching hospitals (Toronto General Hospital, Toronto Western Hospital, the Wellesley Hospital, Sunnybrook and St. Michael's Hospital), with the General and the Western having the lion's share.[17] The students would hear mainly the lectures offered at the General with occasional city-wide rounds bringing them together. Since each hospital could manifestly not offer the full pallette of subspecialties, the arrangement left something to be desired. Nonetheless, as Holmes later said, "It was the glue that held the hospital programs together."[18]

By the 1960s graduate training in radiology meant a program leading to a Royal College fellowship and not to a diploma. As Holmes told the Dean, "Although the training of men for this function [of community radiology] is one of the Department's major responsibilities, it is desirable that we attract a greater number who are interested in an academic career."[19] Holmes scorned what he called "diploma course thinking," as distinct from "fellowship thinking." "In the era of 'Diploma Course Thinking' a man was attached to a service department, received some casual supervision and a few lectures, and he was left to shift for himself to too great a degree. In the new 'Fellowship Thinking' the Faculty will be obliged to upgrade their attitude." The emphasis would be on "academic effort" not "service load."[20] The diploma course was abolished in 1972.

Interns and Residents

But let's not get ahead of our story. From the beginning, the bulk of training would be done in internships and residencies whether linked to the diploma program or not. This story began at the Toronto General Hospital. What was Richards to do for the annual salary of $300 that he received from the Faculty of Medicine? From the very beginning TGH assumed the responsibility of training interns and residents, or "housemen," in radiology. In 1922 we find the hospital's medical advisory board agreeing to Richards' recommendation "that the X-Ray Department should be placed upon the list of Services taking House-men in rotation."[21] At that point the service seems to have begun taking on clerks and interns. In 1925 Richards appointed his first resident, the above-mentioned Omer Hague, as a houseman who would spend full-time on the service.[22] These were the years, one recalls, in which Richards was flexing his own muscles, laying down rules for the hospital in using the service, and rejecting dictates about procedures from the surgeons in particular.[23] As part of this campaign, in 1934 his title was changed from associate to associate professor.

Hague was not succeeded by a second resident. Only in 1934 did "senior interns," or residents, start being named regularly in the department of radiology. In that year Frederick N. Blackwell was appointed for two years, Charles D. Hess for one.[24] (Blackwell went off to general practice in Cobourg, ultimately becoming coroner there; Hess became a radiologist at St. Joseph's Hospital in Hamilton.) Over the years ahead, in recruiting people for radiology the department stressed that it was looking for the cream of the crop, not for the GP material found in the diploma program. For example, in 1954, Singleton requested the re-establishment of rotating junior interns in diagnostic radiology: "He was interested in getting the right type of men to go into Radiology," the minutes of the meeting noted. (Singleton was agreeable to giving the junior intern "night duty on some other service," an arresting comment on what was expected of junior physicians in those days.[25])

For decades, the General would bear a reputation as an inhospitable place for residents. As a 1957 report on the "interne shortage" at the hospital commented, "An unfriendly attitude is said to be abroad in this Hospital that is said to be partly on the part of the teaching Staff.... Dissatisfaction with many Administrative matters is commonly discussed."[26] Did Radiology share in this? Said one report on the department, "The format of Grand Rounds to many residents is deficient in that there appears to be a sotto voce dialogue between the interrogator from the staff and the resident from the platform." "Greater freedom of discussion" between staff and residents "with an easier incorporation of resident opinions" was thought desirable.[27] As the oldest site for training radiologists in Toronto, TGH had thus accumulated its share of problems as well as triumphs.

Meanwhile at the Hospital for Sick Children education in radiology for undergraduates flourished while that for graduates languished. As early as 1922, Rolph was giving "Lectures in Radiology as applied to children...to the students of the Fifth Year of University throughout the term, as well as a brief series comprising a part of the Summer post-graduate course in Paediatrics."[28] Yet despite Rolph's appointment as "clinician," before the Second World War the hospital department of radiology had no systematic relationship with the university. It was not a teaching department, in other words, despite the recommendation of the Johns Hopkins professor Lewellys Barker in 1930 that hospital and university come together.[29] In 1927 Rolph was granted "assistant demonstrator" status at the university (senior demonstrator after 1930). Yet, unlike Richards, he never achieved professor status.

Radiology at HSC got its first "intern" in 1945, just at the end of the Rolph years. By "intern," resident is presumably meant, young physicians just out of the army who had enrolled in the diploma program.[30] In October of that year Dr. William Sloan from TGH rotated through the service for two months. (Sloan would become a distinguished radiologist at Shaughnessy Hospital in Vancouver.[31]) Seven months later John Munn came on staff as assistant radiologist. The first resident under Munn—rotating, of course, like all residents at HSC—was Owen Millar, later a well-known pediatric radiologist and radiotherapist. Munn immediately began teaching in the diploma program, and prided himself as having trained more than a hundred of its graduates over the years.[32] When in the academic year 1948-49 Munn was granted the university rank of associate, radiology at HSC officially became a university department, though this recognition was a bit belated given that teaching had been going on since at least the First World War and maybe before.[33] (St. Michael's, the Western and Sunnybrook also simultaneously became university departments.) In 1948 as well, the Council of the Royal College approved HSC for graduate training in radiology.[34] Therefore 1948-49 is the academic year in which postgraduate training at HSC really got going. In November 1948 Alan Brown, the professor of pediatrics, recommended the definitive move: "that the Department of Radiology of this hospital cooperate in plans for a University Post Graduate course in radiology."[35]

Yet a systematic program of postgraduate education in radiology at HSC began only after 1967 under Bernard Reilly. He initiated radiology rounds for the residents, as well as persuading them to attend the rounds of other departments and to give papers at meetings. As HSC radiologist Frederic Moes recalled, "It was radiology on a higher level than it had been in every aspect." "Everything was encouraged for teaching. The integration between radiology and the clinical departments was encouraged. For a long time, in whatever ward you happened to be doing x-rays for, the interns came down from that ward at 2:00 every day and you went over films with them." Reilly encouraged the writing of papers. "If you were interested in doing something he would always say fine, go ahead."[36] Under Reilly, pediatric radiology was taught systematically to the undergraduates, each of the six staff radiologists taking four sessions of eight to ten students.[37] The Reilly years thus marked the blossoming of education in radiology at the children's hospital.

In contrast to the General and the Hospital for Sick Children, training in radiology began late in time at Toronto's other teaching hospitals. Next came St. Michael's Hospital. Eugene Shannon had been appointed to the university department of radiology in 1948, at the same time as Munn. In that year SMH had been certified by the Royal College for training, again at the same time as Sick Kids. Yet nothing actually happened at St. Mike's for the next seven years. In October 1955, at a meeting of the medical advisory board, W. K. Welsh observed, that Shannon had signed a contract to be full-time radiologist and "that people should be able to train here in radiology, both therapeutic and diagnostic."[38] When Bruce Bird took over the department in 1963, there was one resident. Accordingly, radiology training at St. Mike's was essentially a post-1960s phenomenon.

If St. Mike's got into teaching belatedly and rather unwillingly, Mount Sinai Hospital jumped in early and enthusiastically, limited only by resources rather than desire. Yet there was an urgency about this that went beyond enthusiam for learning, though that was present too. Although Jewish high school students were not discriminated against in entering medical school (until after World War II, all qualified graduates automatically had the right of medical-school admission), Jewish medical graduates were discriminated against in their application for residencies in the specialties. A Jewish teaching hospital was therefore considered essential. As Mt. Sinai administrator Sidney Liswood put it much later in 1962 to Dean John Hamilton, once previous discrimination had begun to fade, "Since we are the only public general hospital under Jewish auspices in Metropolitan Toronto, the pressure on us for staff appointments by Jewish physicians is extremely great, and in fact, greater than we have room for on our staff."[39]

It is thus understandable why the board of directors made it absolutely clear in the late 1940s, as the New Mount Sinai Hospital on University Avenue was being planned, that teaching was important to them. In 1947 their planning consultant, Dr. J. J. Golub, told them the hospital would have to negotiate with the university for an affiliation, "so that undergraduate, graduate and postgraduate teaching would be carried on under the auspices of the University and research can be carried on in the hospital.... The

University demands that the facilities be suitable and that the medical staff be of the calibre to be qualified for teaching students. The hospital, on the other hand, insists that the staff be given rank in the University providing the doctors are qualifed." Among necessary facilities, said Golub, the university would want "X-ray laboratories."[40] Just after opening in 1953, the hospital determined it would need a resident in radiology for the sake of postgraduate accreditation (which it obtained in 1955).[41] So there was clearly institutional will from the beginning.

Yet the biggest factor moving the Sinai into medical education was Bernie Shapiro's own enthusiasm for teaching. In the fall of 1955, shortly after coming to the hospital, he described his sessions with the interns. "Every Friday afternoon we devote ourselves to the Interne Group of the Hospital. The Internes, as many as are free, come to my office and we discuss the interesting cases that have passed through the department during the past week.... These usually last for an hour or an hour and a half, depending on the degree of interest and the amount of discussion that the various cases arouse. These conferences are informal and anyone can interrupt at any time and ask as many questions as they desire."[42] As for postgraduate teaching, the Sinai shortly got Royal College approval for training in radiology. In September 1962 the Sinai formally became a university teaching hospital as the Department of Medicine was certified as a teaching department.[43] In the academic year 1967-68, radiology formally became a teaching department with Shapiro's appointment to the Faculty of Medicine.[44] By 1986 the radiology department of the Mount Sinai was averaging around eight residents a year, putting it in the mid-range of the Toronto teaching hospitals.

The development of radiology training at Toronto's other hospitals is considered in connection with other aspects of their history.

Royal College Certification

Although the history of certification in radiology is essentially a national rather than a Toronto story, changes in certification did affect the development of radiology in Toronto. The certification narrative also places the local story in context, for Toronto and English Canada as a whole have always been buffeted in a very powerful cross-draft between Britain and the United States. Developments in Britain heavily influenced the whole ethos of advanced training in Canada, as the Royal College of Physicians and Surgeons, incorporated by an Act of Parliament in 1929, for decades saw itself as profoundly British in spirit. For example, in 1931 it sought recognition by the General Medical Council of Great Britain and begged the King to act as Patron of the College.[45]

Yet it was the drive for specialism in the United States in the 1930s to which the Royal College of Canada responded with its own push toward certification and fellowship examinations in the various disciplines. In 1934, a specialty Board was created for radiology in the United States. It was in these years that events began to unfold in Canada as well. Toronto, of course, had always danced in this great tug-of-war for influence between America and Britain. In training, bearing and orientation, Richards and Ash were British to the core. Yet many of the early radiologists, such as William H. Dickson and John Munn, had trained in the United States.

Curiously, radiology triggered the drive toward specialism of the Royal College in Canada. In 1936 the Section on Radiology of the Canadian Medical Association at its meeting in Victoria proposed "that the Radiologists of Canada establish a Board of Radiology." Later that year W. A. Jones, the professor of radiology at Queen's University and then president of the Canadian Association of Radiologists, suggested that the Royal College might set up such a board. This could be done for other specialties as well. The implication was that if the College did not take over the task of certification, the radiologists would press ahead on their own. In 1937 the College identified twelve branches of medicine as possible specialties for certification, radiology being one. (This was separate from the fellowship exams that one could already sit for medicine and surgery.) On the radiology committee that the College struck in the fall of 1937 sat Jones and Richards.[46] By this time, the Canadian Association of Radiologists had constituted itself as a separate body, and the CAR and the Royal College jointly agreed that certification in radiology would require a three-year residency after internship, plus two more years of practice. In 1942 the certification of radiologists without exam was approved, and the future strategy would be grandfathering in the older radiologists, examining the younger.[47]

As the Second World War came to an end, it became obvious that a fellowship was better. Being a certified specialist was seen as somehow inferior to receiving a fellowship following a rigorous examination. Richards began pressing for a "searching" examination for radiologists that would lead to a fellowship. Following his intervention, in June 1945, the Council of the Royal College voted to include radiology among the specialties suitable for fellowship. Meanwhile the College had been certifying specialists without examination, and by this time there were 130 of them in Canada. (Two of the three names on the list for Toronto were community radiologists; Harry M. Worth of TGH and HSC was the third.[48])

In 1946 the examinations for certification began. The following year it became possible to write in either therapeutic or diagnostic radiology.[49] Finally, in 1948, a fellowship examination in radiology commenced. Two candidates attempted the first exam; neither passed.[50] (Meanwhile, about half were passing the certification exam.) Throughout the 1950s the pressure became stronger and stronger to abolish the specialist certification and go over to a single fellowship examination for all specialties. In 1962 the College finally accepted "a single standard of training." To qualify to write the exam one would have to do a general internship plus four additional years of graduate training.[51] (Later that year the College stipulated that one of the four years would have to be spent training outside of radiology, in medicine, pathology, and so forth.[52])

Taking an activist role to improve quality in the specialties, since 1948 the College had been certifying hospitals for training in radiology. The Toronto General Hospital, St. Michael's Hospital, and the Hospital for Sick Children had all been approved that year (the Toronto Western Hospital in 1949).[53] Then in the mid-1950s the College decided to press for the upgrading of hospital training programs in radiology.[54]

These two trains of events—the steady upgrading of radiology certification into a five-year program leading to a fellowship and the improvement of hospital standards—had repercussions on the training of radiologists in Toronto. Those who had passed the fellowship examination became a kind of local elite. Brian Holmes was the first in Canada in 1952, followed by several others, such as Kenneth Hodge, later chief of radiology at Sunnybrook, in the academic year 1955-56. Having a fellowship exam to aim for increased the role of hospitals, such as the General, as a trainer of elites. Holmes took pride that almost none of the radiology residents from the General who sat College exams from 1950 to 1967 failed. "That meant we were doing something right," he later said. Other Toronto teaching hospitals did not have such good luck.[55] Toronto as a whole became privileged by the critical mass of specialists and fellows in the city who compiled an "underground bank" of questions superior to that found in other centers, thus giving Toronto candidates a leg up.[56]

Another consequence of emphasizing the fellowship exam was to divide the pool of radiology trainees into two clearly defined groups: Those doing only the diploma would march out into the world of general practice. Those "bright young men," as Holmes put it,[57] seeking the fellowship would become full-blooded radiologists. The fellowship program was to be unhooked from the diploma program. In the 1960s it became common for fellowship aspirants not even to aim for the diploma. Since medicine historically has always shunned anything resembling a two-class system, some of whose products would by definition be "second-class," the diploma program became steadily de-emphasized and was abolished in 1972. Radiology would henceforth be an elite specialty.

Integration

The basic problem Toronto faced in the 1960s was the soaring demand for radiologists in the context of a training system that was almost completely uncoordinated. By the late 1940s Toronto had five hospitals with postgraduate teaching programs in radiology: Toronto General Hospital, the Hospital for Sick Children, the Toronto Western Hospital, St. Michael's Hospital, and Sunnybrook Hospital. All were quite unaccustomed to cooperating with one another. As the Dean of the Faculty, A. L. Chute, complained in 1968, "Historically, hospitals were local community projects to meet local needs and supported in large part by donations from public-spirited citizens.... Each had a highly individualistic attitude, competing with other hospitals for staff, facilities, and community support. No *effective, co-ordinated* planning within the University group of hospitals in regard to total regional needs has taken place."[58] The situation was just as bad in radiology as in other disciplines. "Most radiologists were not university-oriented," said Holmes. "They were hospital people." They had little interest in a university-wide program that, they perceived, would inevitably be dominated by the Toronto General Hospital.

Into this tradition of parochialism burst the events of the 1960s. The sheer number of films that had to be read was rising precipitously. "Since moving into the new Department in 1959," Holmes told the TGH medical advisory board, "there has been a 60% increase in the number of examinations as well as a striking increase in the complexity and nature of the work."[59] The radiologists of the 1930s did not have to deal with angiography, isotope scanning, thermography, xeroradiology. Those of the 1960s did.

In addition, the new requirement of the Royal College that one of the four years of specialist training be spent outside of radiology meant that at any time a quarter of the residents would be away. A twenty-five percent increase would be required just to cover the service. Holmes concluded that the graduation of radiologists at the University of Toronto would have to be accelerated from 12 per year to 25.[60]

This need for more radiologists was not just an internal perspective. The public too wanted more radiology, given the miracle stories about angiography and the like that they were reading in the press. "Too Few Radiologists!" blared the *Toronto Star*. "X-ray errors blamed on rush, overwork." "When you're tired and you still have to plough through a lot of work, mistakes happen," Bernard Shapiro of the New Mt. Sinai Hospital was quoted as saying.[61] One in three citizens was having an x-ray every year.[62] The university had to respond.

Thus, these separate teaching hospitals, in their totally uncoordinated residency training programs, began turning out increasing numbers of radiologists. By 1969 there were eight teaching hospitals in diagnostic radiology, the radiology departments of the Wellesley Hospital, the Mount Sinai Hospital, and the Women's College Hospital having recently become teaching departments. These eight departments together had 47 residents: Toronto General 13, Toronto Western 9, St. Michael's 8, Sunnybrook 8, Mount Sinai 8, the Wellesley 1 (Women's College had no residents. Sick Children's was not a home-base for residents but all would rotate through there.[63])

Given these numbers, the status quo was clearly unacceptable. The eight disparate hospital training programs had to be forged into a single university-wide program. Holmes understood this at the outset of taking office. In 1968 he said that the university department should aim at developing a "Toronto University Hospital System" in which the department of radiology would drive forward an increase in staffing across all the hospitals and pay for it from "an academic budget for radiology."[64] As he told the Dean in 1971, "The Department has adopted the policy of converting the various hospital based programmes into a fully integrated University programme aided by a Programme Co-ordinator."[65] In the context of the status quo, this was really quite a revolutionary aspiration.

What had been done previously to coordinate this scatter of hospital programs? Very little. In 1951 Holmes and Harnick triggered the creation of the Toronto Radiological Society. They got the idea from meetings of the New England Roentgen Ray Society they had both attended when they were in Boston as residents. It had met every month at the Harvard Club in Boston. "We liked the way it brought people together from cities around New England." Harnick, who had come from Toronto, told Holmes that in Toronto there had been no such group, earlier attempts shattering because of personality clashes among Richards, Shannon, Kruger, and the other hospital chiefs. "Lou and I thought we could get four young Turks and start a society and make it go," said Holmes. Holmes took the idea to Singleton, then his chief, and Singleton "who was a great enthusiast for things thought it a great idea. And so we managed to put out a call to radiologists at hospitals around Toronto and sometime in '51 we had the first meeting in The Old Lecture Theatre at TGH. There were maybe twenty people in that room."

Not at the University Club? Holmes laughed. "No. We were young people with an idea. Singleton may have been a club member. But I was thirty-one. In fact at that point I had never heard of the University Club."

Singleton was nominated as President of the Toronto Radiological Society, Holmes as secretary. It soon became known as the "Holmes-Harnick Society." As the TRS developed, it would bring in about five speakers a year, and worked as a unifying factor in the community of radiologists.

In the late '50s Holmes tried other experiments in cross-hospital teaching. First he tried organizing slide sessions. As Douglas Sanders recalled, "He had access to enormous teaching materials that had been set aside before 1960 in the basement. He had a collection of his own teaching slides which he had made from the teaching collection at the Mass. General during training. He said if you guys are interested, I'll show them to you on a regular basis. It was on the fourth floor of the Dunlap Building. There was no heat. We did that on a regular basis and before long we collected residents from other places who came when they could."

Next, Holmes instituted an evening "quiz session" for staff radiologists from Toronto. Sanders said, "It was for whenever they could come after supper, and look at half a dozen cases which usually were presented by residents. The residents showed films and gave histories and we all sat in the teaching room and discussed them. It was a unifying factor."[66]

When Holmes was chief of the TGH department and chair of the university department between 1965 and 1973, he tried hard to press forward on unification. By 1971 he had set up a small radiology departmental office on the University of Toronto campus, the purpose of which was, in official language, "the full recognition of the truly academic aspects of the departmental function as opposed to the hospital service function." What Holmes later said was, "I wanted to de-emphasize the dominant role of the TGH and wanted the chairman to be seen as more neutral." The office had a small budget and gave space to the program coordinator.[67] (Only around 1979, however, did Lansdown secure a regular departmental office in the FitzGerald Building.) Indeed, Holmes's conception in these years was exactly that which came to pass much later, namely to be a "professor-chairman" of radiology based at the university, supported by the university and independent of the hospitals.[68]

To de-emphasize further the role of the Toronto General Hospital, Holmes set up a senior advisory committee representing all the hospitals, and made Douglas Sanders the representative of TGH. "When I chaired the meeting, I didn't wear a hospital hat," he said.

Holmes was aided in these efforts by the Royal College's growing efforts to transfer responsibility for postgraduate training from the hospitals to the universities. Throughout the 1960s the Royal College became ever more involved with the Association of Canadian Medical Colleges, and with setting standards for training programs. In 1975 the Royal College finally formally insisted that all postgraduate medical education be supervised by universities and not by hospitals, definitively breaking hospital control of training.[69]

Yet despite the growing punch of the Royal College, and despite his own manifest energy, organizing ability, and leadership skills, Holmes was able to do little during his chairmanship to bring the departmental training programs together. With the exception of the small campus office, during his eight years there was no progress toward forging the eight disparate hospital departments of radiology into a single university department. What explains this puzzling lack of progress?

The problem was that the staff in both the weakest and the strongest departments opposed unification. Under Harnick, radiology at the Toronto Western Hospital had not kept abreast. Harnick had no interest in joining a unified program, and Holmes, because of his long friendship with Harnick, felt reluctant to press the chief at the Western on this matter. "The chiefs at the hospitals like Harnick and Bruce Bird," said Holmes, "were personal friends and colleagues. We wanted to do things together. There was no competition between us. These people had always run independent shows and I was treading on their independence."

But there was also unease at the General at having to rotate one's own interns through hospitals as weak as the Western was reputed to be. Senior radiologists there would say, according to Lansdown, "If you bring this rotation in we'll quit. The TGH felt they had the best training program, the best residents, why should they see their people rotate outwards?"

Caught in a crossfire, Holmes pulled back. During his chairmanship nothing was done about integrating the departmental programs.

When Lansdown became chair of the university department and chief at the General in 1974, he made another go at unification. He was goaded by two kinds of pressures. Positive pressures came from the Royal College and from his program co-ordinator Derek Harwood-Nash at Sick Kids. For example, in 1978, Harwood-Nash centralized all applications for a residency in radiology into a pool. Each hospital would have a first, second and third choice. As well, Harwood-Nash moved to take control of the residency program as a whole, insisting that *all* the rotations be under the supervision of the Program Coordinator, and that all changes, problems, questions and defaults should be referred to me."[70] This authority derived from the new power of the Royal College, and represented a wake-up call to those who thought that integration might simply be put out of mind like a bad dream.

Because some of the hospitals were making special deals with applicants in the pool, when Marvin Steinhardt became program director in 1979, he and Lansdown created a central interviewing committee to let the hospitals bid for applications. The committee would then try to match them.[71]

Another positive force for change was the views of the residents themselves, who were becoming increasingly restive at the status quo. In several surveys residents expressed a desire to see more rotations and get to know radiology outside their home-base hospital.

But there were negative pressures as well. Lansdown was ultimately forced to take action by the growing crisis at the Toronto Western Hospital. It is not as though he had not been forwarned. In 1979 an internal survey sponsored by the university department found that staff were often unavailable to the residents. The residents got little feedback on their reports of films. Appearing throughout the report were such phrases as, "The rheumatology patients are 'private' and not seen to any degree by the residents." Yet in reporting films on public patients, the residents were unsupervised. They found it very hard to get previous films. There were virtually no rotations in the subspecialties, indeed a lack of subspecialization. Surprisingly, on the whole the assessment was upbeat, giving no sense of crisis.[72]

Yet to radiologists at other hospitals it was clear that a crisis was approaching at the Western. "The residents were very, very unhappy with the teaching there," said Bernard Shapiro later. "It was Harnick and his group. They weren't giving them what they were supposed to learn. They didn't spend any time with them. They were never around."[73]

In truth, Lansdown should probably have intervened at this point. But he was Harnick's ex-resident, and felt deferential towards his former chief. "I had met with Harnick over the years," said Lansdown later. "I'd tell him 'I think you should do this. All the other hospitals are.' He'd sit there with his cigar and nod. Here is his ex-resident telling him what to do. 'Yes, um um.'" Thus the problems continued to grow.

In 1982 the residents made their unhappiness manifest. Quizzed in another internal department review, they said they were "exposed only to the 'public' patients and have no interaction with the large 'private' service." The eleven residents interviewed all said that the TWH training program should be disbanded.[74]

This report caused alarm within the university department. Lansdown, chairman of the department, went to Dean Frederick Lowy and recommended that the Western be dropped from the teaching program. Yet both men felt pinioned by the magnitude of the problem. "This is political dynamite," said Lowy.[75] In the meantime Harnick had neglected to communicate the results of the survey to any of his colleagues. The hospital department was sailing blithely into the gathering storm.

The following year, in 1983, the crisis erupted. The Royal College had sent an examiner, Douglas MacEwan, the professor of radiology at the University of Manitoba, to Toronto to conduct an inspection. Although he found the other seven departments acceptable, MacEwan was not pleased at what he found at the Western. Rather than making suggestions solely about the Western, MacEwan recommended that the entire university department of radiology be placed on probation.

Lansdown and Steinhardt went to MacEwan's hotel room and remonstrated. The whole program and not just the Western? MacEwan said, as Lansdown remembers, "No no, we can't do that anymore. This is a university program and so if you have one weak link everything has to go."

Thus, academic radiology at Toronto received a grave slap in the face. The chairs of the other hospital departments were "roaring mad," as Lansdown put it. Lansdown and the Dean went to the officers at the Western. At first they were incredulous. The chairman of the board finally looked at the chief executive officer, "How could this have ever happened?" he asked. The CEO said, "I'm dumbfounded. I didn't realize this."[76] Harnick stepped down. The Western agreed to a massive revitalizing of the radiology department.

Out of the crisis at Toronto Western Hospital a number of positive developments emerged. For one thing, the department at the Western got a dynamic new acting chief, Karel TerBrugge, who swiftly brought the service up to speed. (see p. 164). Another development concerned the university department, for Lansdown was retiring as chair in 1984 after the now standard tenure of ten years. For the first time in its history, the department of radiology looked outside to find a new leader.

Recruiting an outsider was a decision reached by Dean Frederick Lowy. After the Royal College had placed the department on probation, Lowy called in two radiologists from elsewhere—Joachim Burhenne from the University of British Columbia and Richard Greenspan from Yale—to consider what should be done. Both strongly urged that the chair of the department be made independent of the hospitals and that radiology residents rotate across all hospital departments.[77] This gave Lowy the mandate he needed. "Radiology was a good service department," he later said. "But we wanted to boost it academically. So we brought in an outsider. It was my call—and I found money for it in my budget. Also, we had just acquired MRI and we needed an MRI specialist. So we brought in Gordon Potts. He'd just written a book on neuro-MRI."[78]

In 1985 Gordon Potts was fifty-eight years old. Born in Auckland, New Zealand, Potts had received an MB from the University of Otago in 1951, then trained in radiology first in Auckland, then in London. He spent 1955 to 1960 doing postgraduate work in radiology at various English institutions, including University

College Hospital and the Central Middlesex Hospital. It was in the late '50s at Atkinson Morley's Hospital in London and at the National Hospital, Queen Square that he developed his expertise in neuroradiology.

In 1960 Potts crossed the Atlantic to the Neurological Institute of Columbia-Presbyterian Medical Center in New York as a neuroradiologist. One of his first achievements there was to invent, with Juan Taveras, a new somersaulting chair for cerebral pneumography.[79] It became the standard chair for a decade until CT made the procedure obsolete. In 1970 Potts became professor of radiology at the New York Hospital–Cornell Medical Center. In 1985, after almost a quarter of a century in New York, he moved to Toronto to become professor and chairman, department of radiology, and radiologist-in-chief at the Toronto Western Hospital. (In 1990 Potts did agree briefly to become chief of radiology at the newly united departments of the Western and the General, now called "the Toronto Hospital," until Chia-Sing Ho took up this post in August 1991.)

The resistance to a university-wide program, so fierce before, melted with Potts's arrival. What had been so difficult for Lansdown, the insider, was straightforward for Potts. Lansdown and Potts became good friends, and so later Lansdown said, tongue in cheek, "Now it was Gord coming in with, 'This is what I've been told. I don't care what you people think.' He was a stranger. One of the difficulties on my part was that I knew everyone, which was an advantage for stability. But here he was saying, 'We must now do this.'"

Thus it was that Potts transformed the university department. Of the various hospital departments of radiology, five had teaching programs. He folded these five into a single university program. The residents would stay at home-base for their first year, but in the three subsequent years they would rotate freely among all the hospital departments. By 1987-88 the new system was in effect.

Potts tried to organize the university department along organ-system lines. "When I arrived, " said Potts, "a GI radiologist in one hospital wouldn't even know who his counterparts were in other hospitals. There was just no contact."[80] So he revamped the training program on the basis of cardiovascular, respiratory, GI, GU, musculo-skeletal, and neuroradiology. He expressly rejected organizing things on the basis of imaging technology: "Radiologists have to master all the modalities in their organ system, because single modalities are vulnerable to take-over by other specialties. We've seen this in cardiac." These university-wide subspecialty divisions were in place by 1991-92.[81]

Potts solicited feedback from the residents on who was best and worst at teaching. "Then I could go to the hospital chiefs and say, if this can't be corrected we'll have to reduce the number of residents coming to your hospital. So they'd try to strengthen their programs." Potts also initiated an annual refresher course in organ-imaging program to help integrate the faculty and keep them abreast of new advances in radiology.

"Consensus departments are very difficult to re-orient," Potts said modestly. "Sometimes it's necessary to bring in outside blood." With Potts's arrival, century-old Toronto traditions had folded literally overnight. When, in 1991, he handed the chair over to Walter Kucharczyk, he had created a university department of radiology.

Endnotes

[1] Henry K. Pancoast, "Reminiscences of a Radiologist," *AJR*, 39 (1938), pp. 169-186, quote p. 172.

[2] College of Physicians and Surgeons of Ontario, minutes of Council meeting, July 1910, re: "Teaching the Use of X-Rays as Part of Curriculum." In CPSO Archives.

[3] Editorial, "The Future of the Roentgenologist," *Canada Lancet*, 64 (Feb. 1925), pp. 52-53, quote p. 53.

[4] W. A. Jones, "Radiological Education," *CMAJ*, 37 (1937), pp. 480-482.

[5] "Special Committees Book," July 2, 1919. University of Toronto Archives, A86-0027, box 11.

[6] "Special Meeting of the Council of the Faculty of Medicine," Nov. 10, 1919, p. 115. University of Toronto Archives, A86-0027, box 18. "Regular Meeting of the Council....," Dec. 3, 1920, p. 307, where Richards was appointed associate.

[7]"Regular Meeting of the Council of the Faculty of Medicine," Dec. 3, 1920, p. 310, box 18. At a later meeting the Faculty council resolved that radiology should be a "subordinate department," yet not subordinated to any of the clinical departments. Radiology was not apparently subordinated to any other department, for the staff listing of the Faculty for 1921-22 shows it as an independent department. See Faculty Council minutes for Feb. 4, 1921, p. 333; Feb. 3, 1922, p. 425.

[8]Arthur U. Desjardins, "The Status of Radiology in America," *JAMA*, 92 (Mar. 30, 1929), pp. 1035-39, quote p. 1036.

[9]At its meeting of Dec. 2, 1921, the Faculty's Committee on Post Graduate Studies recommended both the short course and the diploma course (pp. 420-421). On the British diploma programs see A. E. Barclay, "The Old Order Changes," *British Journal of Radiology*, 22 (1949), pp. 300-308, esp. p. 305.

[10]Faculty Council, Feb. 3, 1922, p. 440.

[11]"Minutes of Annual Conference between the Medical Faculties of Toronto and McGill Universities, held at McGill University, Mar. 18, 1922," p. 458 (appended to minutes of Faculty council meeting, box 18).

[12]University of Toronto Archives, A79-0023, box 7 (Wil).

[13]On the beginnings of the diploma see W. G. Cosbie, *The Toronto General Hospital, 1819-1965: A Chronicle* (Toronto: Macmillan, 1975), p. 190.

[14]E. T. Kellam, "Presidential Address, 1923-24," CPSO Archives.

[15]University of Toronto, *Report of the Dean of the Faculty of Medicine, session 1965-1966*, p. 103.

[16]*Report of the Dean, 1949-1950*, p. 48.

[17]See "DMR Course, Diagnosis, 1968-1969," list of students, Aug. 26, 1968. In administrative files, Department of Diagnostic Imaging, TTH General Division. In truth, the student body was a mixture, composed of radiology residents as well.

[18]R. Brian Holmes interview of June 3, 1994.

[19]*Report of the Dean, 1965-1966*, p. 103.

[20]"University of Toronto, Future Graduate Training Programmes in Diagnostic Radiology" [March 1968], pp. 5-6. In TTH radiology offices' files.

[21]TGH MAB, Mar. 13, 1922.

[22]TGH MAB, Jan. 27, 1925.

[23]Gordon E. Richards, "X-Rays and Radium in the Management of Breast Carcinoma," *CMAJ*, 16 (1926), pp. 358-366. "There are still a few surgeons who by attempting to dictate their own wishes in these cases only succeed in tying the hands of the man who is being held responsible for the outcome of the treatment, in a manner which no surgeon would tolerate in his own work" (p. 364).

[24]TGH Trustees, Feb. 28, 1934, p. 831.

[25]TGH MAB, Dec. 16, 1954.

[26]TGH MAB, "Report on Interne Shortage" by Donald Wilson et al., attached to minutes of Apr. 18, 1957.

[27]Department of Radiology, "Departmental Survey," 1979, under TGH, p. 4. In Lansdown Papers.

[28]HSC, *Annual Report, 1922*, p. 38.

[29]HSC Trustees, Mar. 25, 1930. The minutes record that, in a letter, "Mr. Barker strongly recommended a close relation between the two institutions."

[30]The term "resident" is first used in HSC's *Annual Reports* in 1951 (p. 6).

[31]HSC MAB, Oct. 13, 1945.

[32]"Meet the Staff, Dr. J. D. Munn," [HSC] *Paediatric Patter,* Apr. 1962, p. 1.

[33]*Report of the Dean, 1948-1949,* p. 43.

[34]RCPS Council, Nov. 25-26, 1948, p. 50.

[35]HSC MAB, Nov. 10, 1948.

[36]Frederic Moes interview, Jan. 11, 1995.

[37]HSC MAB, June 5, 1974.

[38]SMH MAB, Oct. 3, 1955.

[39]MSH, "Conversation with Dr. John Hamilton in His Office on May 1, 1962," a résumé prepared for the executive committee and interfiled with the committee's minutes. Because it was a summary of a previous meeting, Liswood used past tenses, which I have altered to the present.

[40]MSH Directors, Apr. 16, 1947.

[41]MSH Directors, Dec. 10, 1954.

[42]Shapiro report to Board of Directors, Sept. 30, 1955, interfiled with Board minutes.

[43]At the executive committee meeting of June 1, 1962, Sidney Liswood said the university would grant teaching status to the department of medicine as of September.

[44]*Report of the Dean, 1967-68,* p. 130.

[45]RCPS minutes of Council, Nov. 19, 1931, pp. 9, 22. In Archives of RCPS in Ottawa.

[46]This story has been reconstructed from the minutes of the RCPS Council, including June 22, 1936, p. 6; Oct. 31, 1936, pp. 12-16; June 21, 1937, pp. 14-20; Oct. 29-30, 1937, pp. 27-28, 38.

[47]RCPS Council, June 16, 1942, p. 26.

[48]RCPS Council, June 16, 1945, pp. 17-20.

[49]RCPS Council, Nov. 27, 1947, p. 26.

[50]RCPS Council, Nov. 25-26, 1948, p. 20.

[51]RCPS Council, Jan. 15-16, 1962. The requirements were spelled out at the meeting of Sept. 1962.

[52]RCPS, "Regulations Relating to the Training Requirements for the Examinations in Diagnostic Radiology," Sept. 1962. For the impact of this on the Toronto training program see TGH MAB, Oct. 21, 1965.

[53]RCPS Council, Nov. 25-26, 1948, pp. 50-51; June 17-18, 1949, p. 55.

[54]RCPS Council, Oct. 29, 1953, p. 30, re sending out a questionnaire.

[55]Holmes interview.

[56]RCPS, Radiology Committee, June 14, 1988, p. 3.

[57]"University of Toronto, Future Graduate Training Programmes in Diagnostic Radiology," March 1968, p. 6. In departmental files, TTH Department of Diagnostic Imaging.

[58]"Notes Prepared by Dr. A. L. Chute, Dean of Medicine, Setting Forth Major Problems for Consideration. Memorandum 2," Sept. 1, 1968, p. 3. Archives of Ontario, RG 10-0-1913.

[59]Holmes to Wightman, Oct. 12, 1965, attached to TGH MAB, Oct. 21, 1965.

[60]"Planing Document," Mar. 1968, pp. 3-4.

[61]"Too Few Radiologists," *Toronto Star,* Oct. 27, 1969, p. 33.

[62]"Department of Radiology, Presentation to Interdepartmental Planning Co-ordination Committee, Toronto General Hospital," May 25, 1966, p. 28.

[63]"Report of the Independent Planning Committee Constituted by the Faculty Council of the Faculty of Medicine, University of Toronto," Oct. 1, 1969, p. 61. Copy of this found in SMH Archives.

[64]"Future Graduate Training Programmes," 1968, pp. 11-12.

[65]*Report of the Dean, 1970-71*, p. 157.

[66]Douglas Sanders interview, Dec. 28, 1994.

[67]*Report of the Dean, 1970-71*, p. 157.

[68]"Future Graduate Training Programmes," 1968, p. 11.

[69]David A. E. Shephard, *The Royal College of Physicians and Surgeons of Canada, 1960-1980* (Ottawa: RCPS, 1985), pp. 145-147, 199-205.

[70]Derek Harwood-Nash, "Report by Program Coordinator," June 1978, p. 2. In Lansdown Papers.

[71]Lansdown interview, May 17, 1995.

[72]Department of Radiology, "Departmental Survey 1979," section on TWH, pp. 1-2.

[73]Bernard Shapiro interview, Jan. 24, 1995.

[74]"University of Toronto Internal Review of Specialty Programs at Teaching Hospitals," June 18, 1982, found in SMH Archives.

[75]Lansdown interview.

[76]This is in the recollection of Lansdown, who attended the meeting.

[77]Their reports are in "Radiology Review 1983," in Dean's Office.

[78]Frederick Lowy interview of Mar. 10, 1995. See T. H. Newton and D. G. Potts, eds., *Modern Neuroradiology*, 2 vols. (San Anselmo: Clavadel Press, 1983).

[79]D. Gordon Potts and Juan M. Taveras, "A New Somersaulting Chair for Cerebral Pneumography," *AJR*, 92 (1964), pp. 1249-51.

[80]Gordon Potts interview of Feb. 2, 1994.

[81]University of Toronto, Department of Radiology, *Annual Report, 1991-1992*, p. 2.

Chapter Five
Towards Medical Imaging

In the last quarter of the twentieth century the notion of radiology—with its connotation of reading plain films produced by x-rays—was replaced by the concept of medical imaging, with its suggestion of the many different strategies of visualizing the interior of the body and of doing image-guided interventions. In 1994 the Department of Radiology at the University of Toronto became officially the Department of Medical Imaging. This lexic shift mirrored a dramatic change in the nature of the discipline. It also represented a challenge for the leadership: The heads of radiology departments would not only have to integrate all this new technology into decades-old organizations, they would have to drum up ways of paying for it. For the new technology was shockingly expensive and represented the outlay of sums that in health-care economics would previously have been considered hallucinatory. That the university and hospital departments of radiology in Toronto responded well to these challenges gives evidence that the spirit of Richards and Holmes, of Peters and Ash, was still abroad.

Nuclear Medicine

In the story of nuclear medicine in Toronto, the action begins with the physicists and ends, in a manner of speaking, with the psychiatrists, marked in between by a large turf struggle between the internists and the radiologists.

At a meeting of TGH's medical advisory board on February 26, 1948, Gordon Richards announced that "radio-active isotopes will be available within a few months to this hospital." Provisions had to be made. A committee was to be set up consisting of the disciplines concerned, including James Dauphinee from the Department of Medicine (Dauphinee was also the professor of "pathological chemistry," as medical biochemistry was then called).[1] Richards would chair the committee, thus ensuring that the new investigative technology remained in the hands of the department of radiology.

A year later Richards was dead. In 1949 the University and the General Hospital jointly agreed to set up the new "radioactive" lab in the Banting Institute, with Dauphinee as its head. It was to be for the use of all the hospitals. William Paul from the Department of Physics was to coordinate the actual use of the isotopes.[2] This heavy involvement of medicine was actually quite appropriate given the knowledge of the time. An important use of isotopes in the 1950s was therapeutic, involving thyroid cancer and multiple myeloma, and isotope therapy lay really in the province of endocrinology. Yet isotopes were used as tracers as well, and with Richards' death the radiologists had been virtually switched out. When in 1953 K. J. R. ("Kager") Wightman of the Department of Medicine recommended that TGH set up an istopes lab in the new building, he stated firmly, "The radio-isotope laboratory should *not* be associated with the Radiology Department."[3] By 1955 there were two isotope committees on the scene: a university one chaired by Dauphinee, and a TGH committee chaired by Wightman. Both men of course were internists.[4]

Technologic change soon put radiology back in the picture, however. The development of the gamma camera—most notably a model that Hal Anger invented in 1957—meant that radioactive thyroid scans and the like could be imaged, not just followed with a scintillation scanner or counter.[5] At this point radioisotope diagnosis and therapy began to take off. In the late 1950s Bill Paul organized a one-week course on the biology of nuclear medicine. "It was so well-recognized," said Bernie Shapiro, "that until we set up the Royal College course, people accepted it as evidence of quality if somebody applied for a [nuclear-medicine] license."[6] TGH got its first gamma camera around 1966. At that time Donald

Wood of the Department of Medicine began a lecture course on nuclear medicine that was inserted into the radiology training program. (The radiology residents had been lamenting that they got no training in radioisotopes for diagnosis, and that it was a requirement of the American Board.[7])

So rapidly was the nuclear medicine program growing at TGH that it required new space. In 1968 the Board decided to move forward with a radioactive isotope laboratory, to be placed in the Burnside Building.[8] Thanks to Holmes's relentless politicking, in 1970 the hospital decided to place the new Division of Nuclear Medicine within the newly created Department of Radiological Sciences.[9] The internist Donald Wood would head the divison, but overall control would be under radiology. Second in command to Wood was the young David Gilday, a McGill graduate (1966) who had just finished a radiology residency at Winnipeg General Hospital in 1970. He too arrived in July 1970, and was joined the next year by internist Shirley Murray from Women's College Hospital.

These arrangements led, unfortunately, to anything except stability. The Burnside Building turned out to be unsuitable, and the division began searching frantically for new quarters. The Royal College declared the division's training program to be virtually non-existent and threatened disqualification. Wood resigned. Gilday stayed on for a bit as acting director, then left the General to become head of the new nuclear medicine program at Sick Kids. It was at this point Ted Lansdown, as the new chair of the department, held the troubled division together by finding new space and searching for a new head. After a hiatus, David Feiglin (Melbourne MB 1967) became director of "Nukes" at TGH in March 1976 . This initiated a period of stability which continued into the early 1990s under Sylvain Houle (see p. 152). The story of nuclear medicine at the General in these years illustrates the underlying force of the image theme: as soon as medical data become images, they tend to revert to radiology. (Exceptions to this are coronary angiography, cardiac nuclear medicine, and some applications of ultrasound.)

It is unnecessary to trace the development of nuclear medicine at the other seven hospitals in detail. A few high points may be mentioned. The Hospital for Sick Children kept pace virtually step-by-step with the General. The hospital had founded an isotope committee in 1956 to draw upon the lab in the Banting Institute.[10] The committee, run by non-radiologists, dithered. Finally in 1966 radiologist Frederic Moes declared an "urgent need for a separate Isotope Unit" for the hospital itself. The cost was intimidating. A gamma camera, or scintillation camera, alone cost $30,000, to say nothing of the centrifuges, monitoring equipment and the like.[11] There was further delay. Finally in 1969 the hospital decided to share in TGH's isotope lab, with Wood to be cross-appointed to the department of medicine at Sick Kids.[12] It quickly became apparent that this arrangement meant merely sharing expenses rather than a true joint operation and HSC decided to set up its own laboratory in nuclear medicine.[13] In 1972 the hospital recruited Gilday from the General to run the department of radiology's new division of nuclear medicine.[14] The division acquired its first gamma camera the following year, a highly unsatisfactory one in Shapiro's recollection, requiring "very high doses" of isotope. Then, late in 1974, the Women's Auxiliary Centennial Foundation donated a brand new gamma camera. "Camera christenings," noted a captioned photograph of the occasion, "differ from ship christenings in that one does not smash the champagne bottle before it has been emptied."[15]

At the New Mount Sinai Hospital, Shapiro began a nuclear-medicine program in 1965, yet without a full-scale facility for the hospital. Shapiro wanted to expand the program rapidly. In 1967 he appointed Leonard Rosenthall as a temporary consultant in the radiology department's group on nuclear medicine,[16] then encouraged Rosenthall to go and study in England (from which stay Rosenthall, a McGill graduate, returned to the Montreal General Hospital). Next Shapiro appointed the young N. David Greyson, a University of Toronto graduate in 1965 who had just completed a radiology residency. In 1972 Greyson was appointed to Mount Sinai and obtained in the following year the diploma of the American Board of Nuclear Medicine. In 1976 the hospital established a formal division of nuclear medicine with Greyson at its head. At the time that Greyson left the Sinai in 1981 in a dispute about outside income, the division numbered five medical staff, making it the largest nuclear-medicine service in the city. Shapiro himself was for many years Mr. Nuclear Medicine in Canada, being in 1971 a founding member of the Canadian Association of Nuclear Medicine, and in 1976 the first examiner in the subject for the Royal College.

When Greyson left the Sinai in 1981, he became chief of the department of nuclear medicine of St. Michael's Hospital. The internist H. Patrick Higgins had introduced nuclear medicine to SMH in 1956 as he returned from a period of study in England. The division employed one technologist to use a scintillation counter for thyroid uptakes. In a display of farsightedness, in 1966 the hospital purchased a gamma camera, making it the second in the city to have one (after St. Joseph's Hospital), for indeed these much more expensive cameras were to displace the rectilinear scanners that most hospital nuclear-medicine services had previously acquired. When internist William Singer took over the division in 1976, he changed the name from "radioisotope laboratory" to Department of Nuclear Medicine. And it was this already well-equipped service, then, that radiologist Greyson became chief of in 1981.[17] (In 1994 Greyson became chief of the entire department of radiology at St. Mike's.)

At the Toronto Western Hospital, nuclear medicine was separated entirely from radiology. Harnick, dubious about anything that didn't involve x-rays, was skeptical of it and left it to others to establish.[18]

A more recent chapter in the history of nuclear medicine in Toronto involved psychiatry. When the value of positron emission tomography was recognized in the mid-1970s, Toronto radiologists were avid to acquire a cyclotron and a scanner for one of the teaching hospitals. Led by Ted Lansdown, a group came together in 1975 to explore the subject. Because of a lack of funds and of clinical indifference, the group got nowhere.[19]

In 1979 the same persons tried again. At a meeting chaired by neurosurgeon Alan Hudson, the researchers declared the PET scan to be a splendid research instrument, also possessing clinical applications. One should be acquired under the auspices of the division of nuclear medicine of the university radiology department. Again, the steering committee that arose from this meeting got nowhere.[20] But it is interesting that this assemblage of very high-powered senior researchers included an intern at the Toronto General Hospital. The intern was Sylvain Houle.

Houle was the only member of the group actually to have worked with a cyclotron, at the facility in Orsay, France. Born in 1949 in Trois-Rivières, Quebec, Houle had an undergraduate degree in physics and an MSc in electrical engineering from Laval University. At the University of Toronto he studied biomedical engineering with Michael Joy (who had come close to inventing a new gamma camera), simultaneously going to medical school. Houle earned both his MD and his PhD in 1979, just before this strategic meeting on PET took place. He did a residency in radiology and nuclear medicine, becoming FRCP in 1982, and with these highly desirable credentials immediately became cross-appointed between the departments of medicine (nuclear cardiology laboratory) and radiology (division of nuclear medicine) at the Toronto General Hospital. In 1983 he became head of nuclear medicine at TGH. Thus for ten years the young clinician and researcher was a major figure in this youthful science in Toronto.

Meanwhile senior scientific figures in Toronto continued their unsuccessful campaign to raise the seven or eight million dollars involved in the purchase of a cyclotron and the erection of a PET Center. McMaster University in Hamilton, Ontario, had acquired one, and the scientists in Toronto were becoming ever more anxious. Finally, around 1986 Gordon Potts had a chance conversation with Vivian Rakoff, the chair of psychiatry, a man known for his deep humanism and his excellent political connections. They fell to discussing PET scanning. "I told Rakoff the real application of it is in the brain," said Potts later. "The hot area in the next decade is going to be psychiatric diseases rather than tumors."[21] Rakoff, a psychoanalyst, had never in the past shown a great interest in brain biology. Yet he now decided that action was needed if Toronto were to keep ahead of the curve. "He was quite committed to bringing new technology to Toronto," said Houle.[22]

Rakoff went to the provincial government and by April 1987 convinced them to appropriate $7.5 million dollars for a PET scanner for Toronto. Houle and Philip Seeman, a PhD neuroscientist at the Clarke Institute of Psychiatry who had cloned the genes for several dopamine receptors, wrote the brief supporting Rakoff's application. The PET scanner would be situated in a specially constructed PET Centre at the Clarke. Houle would be the director. In February 1993 the PET Centre opened, equipped with a GEMS brain scanner and a 17-MeV cyclotron. It was thus a research institute in psychiatry and not a general hospital that had acquired the latest in nuclear medicine. Houle retained his appointment in radiology, but took up a full-time post amidst the psychiatrists.

It is ironical that Toronto's radiologists had spent forty years trying to gain control of nuclear medicine, only to see it begin to seep away as the skirmish lines of science ranged forward.

Ultrasound

Ultrasound was the next imaging technique to rush on stage. Like nuclear medicine, it threatened at first to evade radiology, then became securely captured. In the late 1960s and early '70s it was among obstetricians and cardiologists that the new technology first spread. In Toronto, radiologists were often resistant.

Ultrasound arrived in Toronto first at the Mount Sinai Hospital. Bernie Shapiro spent three weeks in New York in 1969 checking over the equipment, then decided the hospital should get involved with it. "We took on Murray Miskin," Shapiro said. "We told him he had to do ultrasound. He was unhappy with that because it was very crude then. But we started doing it." When they moved into new quarters in 1974, they relegated Miskin and his equipment to a post-operative room that had eight beds in it. "You can see what happened...," Shapiro trailed off. Demand for the new technology exploded, especially among the cardiologists. Miskin ended up sharing the echocardiology equipment with cardiology, and a fierce turf struggle erupted.

Meanwhile at Toronto General Hospital Ted Lansdown had just been made chief. He had begun an ultrasound service at the St. Boniface Hospital in Winnipeg, making it one of the first centers in Canada to acquire the new technology. One of his preconditions in coming to Toronto was that the General get ultrasound. "So I came here with, 'Oh isn't it great you think ultrasound is worthwhile.'

"Six months after I arrived, the CEO said you know we haven't got enough money for this ultrasound bit. I realized then that I was dealing with sharp businessmen, and that shaking hands or talking about it didn't mean anything." But the obstetricians at the General were very keen to get ultrasound. They proposed sharing a unit with radiology, as did the cardiologists. Gerald Burrow was then the head of medicine. "Burrow came to see me and I told him the story about Miskin. Burrow said fifty-fifty. We'll split it." Income reflecting the activity of both cardiologists and radiologists would be evenly divided. The point is that this new technology, like many of the others, was at first up for grabs among various services. It was not predestined that radiology monopolize it, and if in the end the radiologists did end up doing most of the ultrasound at the General (except for cardiology), it was mainly because they established that they could read the hard-copy films and videotapes better than other specialists. It also had something to do with the arrival at TGH of Stephanie Wilson in 1984, the vigorous young head of the ultrasound section.

By the late 1970s the pressure on other hospitals to acquire ultrasound was tremendous. As the Royal College put it in 1975, "This is currently the most rapidly expanding of the imaging techniques."[23] By 1977 it was established at the Sinai, Sunnybrook, and the General. Hospitals like St. Michael's, already under great financial strain—and pressured as well to acquire CT scanning—, felt that with ultrasound they were looking at an oncoming train. The minutes of one meeting read: "Dr. _____ stated that he couldn't predict where the money would come from to pay for Ultra Sound facilities as money cannot be obtained from the Ministry for expanded services at the present time. It would have to come through the Radiology budget with possible support coming from Obstetrics, Cardiology and General Surgery. He stated that the operating costs would be the most expensive...."

Radiologist Ronald McCallum who attended the meeting shot back, "The priority for Ultra Sound is high. It is urgent that we get the money soon and space must be located.... The Department of Radiology must have updated CAT scanning as well as abdominal Ultra Sound."[24] In 1980 the radiologists at St. Michael's Hospital pushed through an ultrasound service against this kind of resistance. There as elsewhere cardiac ultrasound remained apart.

Because Louis Harnick thought poorly of ultrasound, radiology at the Toronto Western Hospital had little involvement with it until his chiefship ended in 1985. "He missed the boat on ultrasound," said one colleague. "He thought it had no future."[25] Noted a committee reviewing the Western in 1979 somewhat dolefully, "It would seem that there is a lack of ultrasound correlation. The acquisition of an excellent CT scanner in the department has led to almost complete dependence on this modality.... Obstetricians and cardiologists are probably performing an excellent job. However both of these specialties are not sufficiently interested in general abdominal ultrasound. This deficiency should be picked up by the Department of Radiology."[26]

It is unnecessary to rehearse further the experience with ultrasound of individual hospital departments in order to grasp the main point: That bringing ultrasound successfully under the roof of radiology involved leadership, and that at some institutions this was more successful than at others. The term "successful" does not imply empire-building on the part of radiology. It made sense in terms of medical economics as well as professional acumen to center ultrasound in radiology departments rather than elsewhere, because radiology is the one discipline that does not self-refer.

CT and MR Scanning

Few discoveries pointed the way to medical imaging as emphatically as did Computerized Tomography and Magnetic Resonance scanning. Yet, stunning though the clinical results of the new technology were, the costs were staggering in comparison to the previous order of magnitude of radiology equipment. Acquiring CT and MR took great reservoirs of political will and leadership. Negotiating with anxious hospital boards, parsimonious ministries, and jealous rival hospitals demanded executive ability and skill in human relations. It was in these areas that the hospital chiefs in the 1970s and '80s had their mettle tested.

The story goes back to the late 1960s work of the English engineer Godfrey Hounsfield, an employee of the Central Research Laboratories of Electric & Musical Industries Ltd. (EMI) in Middlesex. He was experimenting with computerizing images of sections of the human brain.[27] In April 1972, his new device was announced at a scientific congress in England,[28] and in November of that year the "EMI scanner" was presented for the first time to a large North American audience at the meeting of the Radiological Society of North America (RSNA) at Chicago's Palmer House. (Hounsfield presented his scanner for the first time in the United States at a refresher course at Albert Einstein College of Medicine in New York some months before the RSNA.[29])

Holmes was on the board of directors of the RSNA at the time and had gone down to Chicago a couple of days before the meeting started.[30] "I got in and saw the exhibits before the general membership. And I saw this thing on a Sunday morning. Harnick had come down Saturday night, and he and I saw it together. I got pretty excited and went back to my hotel room and phoned George Wortzman in Toronto. His wife answered the phone and I said is George there because I want him to come to Chicago to see this thing." Mrs. Wortzman replied that her husband was already in Chicago, staying on the fourteenth floor of the Palmer House.

Gloria Wortzman later told Holmes, "You were so excited, you then said, 'Is Charlie Hollenberg there?'" (Hollenberg was head of medicine at the General.)

Holmes, Harnick and Wortzman were very impressed with the CT scanner, as was the rest of the meeting. The session at which Hounsfield and clinician James Ambrose introduced their device was packed.[31] Holmes struck up a conversation with Hounsfield, "a very interesting old-fashioned, bachelor-type scientist Englishman." "I persuaded him that Toronto was on the flight path from Chicago back to London, England."

Hounsfield brought with him to Toronto a video he had made of the scanner in operation. Holmes convened in Toronto a meeting of senior administrators and faculty members to screen the video. He wanted to show it to them, he later said, "because I couldn't believe what I was seeing." Hounsfield ran the video and, said Holmes, "Everybody immediately saw the potential that I saw."

Holmes now contacted Granger Reid in the Ministry of Health, an MD adviser to the minister. "We knew the scanner cost a third of a million dollars but everybody was convinced we had to get this thing right away in Toronto." Reid assigned a couple of Ministry of Health officials to inquire into the scanner to convince himself the Faculty wasn't exaggerating.

A week later Reid told Holmes, as Holmes recalled it, "If you can find a third of the cost, we'll find the other two-thirds." In July 1973 the TGH board of governors approved the purchase of an EMI scanner on the basis proposed by the ministry. A $100,000 bequest from the estate of *Toronto Star* fashion editor Gwen Cowley paid the hospital's share.[32] Holmes and Wortzman were thus the point people moving the project forward, Holmes in the last days of his chiefship and Wortzman as the leading neuroradiologist.

Much later Holmes said to the author, "In some ways Lou Harnick gets a bad rap in your story. And I want to point out that, with the cost of this thing, it was obvious that Toronto would only ever be able to get one. At a meeting of the Senior Committee, Lou

Harnick supported me by saying, in front of all the other hospital chiefs, 'There should be one in Toronto, and it should be at the General Hospital.'" Holmes resumed, "You could almost say the story wouldn't have happened the way it did if it hadn't been for Lou Harnick supporting a single scanner in a central location."

The proviso was that all the other hospitals would have access to it. Holmes set up a user's committee with George Wortzman as the senior neuroradiologist at the General chairing it (the first generation of CTs did head scans only). The other hospital chief neuroradiologists were members. "George was a completely honest, straightforward guy. So the bookings for that thing included people from the other hospitals."

When in May 1974 the General unveiled its new CT scanner, it was the second in Ontario (McMaster University conjointly with Hamilton Civic Hospital had the first in Ontario; the Montreal Neurological Institute had the first in Canada). The hospital gave a big reception, at which Holmes tried to persaude Frank Miller, provincial minister of health, to climb up on the scanner. Miller did so and the press, said Holmes, "took pictures of him lying there with his head in this big gantry. What I did then was pull out a tracing from earlier of somebody's head. I said to him in front of all the press, 'Well, Mr. Minister, you didn't realize it at the time but we had the machine turned on. We have a tracing of your brain, and it gives the report that you have an I. Q. of 190.'"

Miller didn't miss a beat. "This is just great," he said, "because I had my I. Q. done by traditional methods a couple of weeks ago and it was only 170."

Yet while all this banter was going on the radiologists were peering excitedly at the new technology. Sanders said, "Lightbulbs were flashing all over the place. Everbody was saying, how soon can we get access to this. Now we can do all this stuff and don't have to submit patients to the kinds of investigative work that we have been doing [meaning pneumoencephalograms in particular]."

Underutilization was not a problem. By October 1976 there was a backlog of three months.[33] In the meantime Lansdown had become chief and his most urgent priority was securing a second scanner for the General, a total body scanner. Two years of provincial politics deadlocked this plan because other hospitals had meanwhile put in their claims. Also, the fearful costs were making everyone leery. Lansdown, his temper not improved by the fact that, for political reasons the small city of Thunder Bay had just been authorized a CT scanner, finally went to see the deputy minister of health in private. He bluffed the official by saying that TGH was going to put a body scanner in the Medical Arts Building.

"You can't do that with the way things are set up," said the deputy minister. "Legislation hasn't been passed. It's dangerous." (CT wasn't dangerous, said Lansdown, the ministry just wanted to control it.)

Lansdown said, "We have a tertiary hospital with a waiting list of three months of people. We're not really serving our patients well. In fact, desperately poorly. When we hold our press conference and explain to the media and then the public why we are doing this, we think they would approve."

The deputy minister said, "You guys wouldn't do this, would you?"

Lansdown said, "That's the only way we have to go, being overrun and seeing people mistreated."

The deputy minister said, "The scanner in Thunder Bay wasn't my idea."

In 1978 TGH got its second CT scanner, the long-coveted total body scanner.

By this time the other teaching hospitals were exerting great pressure to get scanners of their own. In 1975 St. Michael's Hospital acquired the second CT scanner in Toronto. It was the first total body scanner in Canada. Funded mainly from the hospital's own budget (plus a gift from the Branscombe family), the "Acta-Scanner" was a "first-generation" device with a scanning time of around five minutes and poor resolution.[34] So rapid was the cycle of technologic change in scanning that two years later second-generation scanners with a thirty-second scanning time had already outdated it. Fortunately it could be updated for a mere $200,000. If we wait a month, the medical advisory board was told, the cost will be more than double. It was by now 1977 and the waiting time for the SMH scanner was two months.[35] One can understand the courage required for a hospital already under tremendous financial pressure to make these decisions: The cost of updating the scanner in 1978 amounted to more than the hospital's entire equipment budget.[36]

In time, of course, almost all the other teaching hospitals acquired CT scanners as well. By 1993 the Toronto General Division of the Toronto Hospital had two, the Toronto Western Division two; Sunnybrook, St. Michael's Hospital and the Hospital for Sick Children had two apiece, the Mount Sinai and the Wellesley one apiece, and Women's College Hospital none.[37]

As a footnote to the CT story, Toronto retained a warm spot in its heart for Godfrey Hounsfield, giving him a Gairdner Foundation award in 1976. It was said that Gairdner winners often later received Nobel Prizes (indeed by 1976, eleven of them had done so), and in 1979 Hounsfield received a Nobel as well.

Paying for CT scanning was bad enough. Yet within a decade MR scanning also came along, a true index of the commitment of the Toronto teaching hospitals to keeping abreast of science. This was a time when provincial help had become unreliable and many of the hospitals themselves were deep in debt. It is perhaps these circumstances that help explain Toronto's relative delay in becoming involved with MR. Commercial models were available as early as 1980. When in November 1983 an ad hoc committee of the Toronto General Hospital headed by senior administrator Wanda Plachta recommended moving ahead, Princess Margaret Hospital in Toronto and two hospitals in London, Ontario, already had MR scanners.[38] The cost would be a cool two million dollars plus installation expenses. The government would help out on annual operating costs and some of the installation costs, but the hospital itself would have to pony up the capital expense. So perhaps it was for that reason that, by the spring of 1984, TGH was very receptive to hearing Dean Fred Lowy talk about sharing a unit among the three University Avenue teaching hospitals: the General, the Sinai, and Sick Kids. (In 1982 Lansdown had begun exploratory talks among the three hospitals.) There might even be a second MR scanner. The search committee for the new chair of radiology to replace Ted Lansdown was already interviewing Gordon Potts. Potts was an internationally known MR expert and said he would be very sympathetic to seeing an MR imager in Toronto were he to come here.[39] Where better to put this second imager, in addition to that already promised the tri-hospitals, than at the Toronto Western Hospital. That would simultaneously give a boost to the battered radiology department of that institution, and give Potts a clinical and research base elsewhere than the General. It must have been that logic that led Lowy's committee to recommend definitively in September 1984 that a clinical MR scanner go to the University Avenue hospitals (the "tri-hospitals"), and a small-bore research scanner, funded by the university, go to the Toronto Western Hospital.[40]

The hospitals had to pay for the clinical scanners themselves, and the costs were a bitter pill. The General, for example, had been running a budget shortfall of about $4 million.[41] Radiology was now to absorb about two-thirds of TGH's "high tech" budget.[42] These sums are interesting as a talisman of the power of these departments of radiology within overall hospital life.

In 1986 the tri-hospital MR centre, construction still underway, hired a junior neuroradiologist to run the facility: the thirty-one-year-old Walter Kucharczyk. Kucharczyk was in many ways a counter-pendant to another rising star, the young Sylvain Houle who went on in nuclear medicine. Both had graduated MD from the University of Toronto in 1979. Whereas Houle had trained in France, Kucharczyk had turned south to the United States. After finishing a residency in radiology in Toronto, Kucharczyk had fellowed in MR in neuroradiology at the University of California at San Francisco, then in 1985-86 served as director of the MR center there before returning to Toronto. (It was in 1984 that Houle at age thirty-five became director of nuclear medicine at the Toronto General Hospital.) The parallels are interesting as an indication that a young field draws young talent. In 1991 Kuchar-czyk became chair of the department of radiology of the University of Toronto.

On February 10, 1987, the Tri-hospital Magnetic Resonance Centre opened in a specially-prepared site in the Mulock-Larkin Wing of the Toronto Hospital. Health Minister Murray Elston attended the ceremony and praised the new co-operativeness of the Toronto teaching hospitals.[43] It was in many ways the beginning of a new era.

Interventional Radiology

Finally, radiology shaded into medical imaging by getting away from the interpretation of images to the performance of procedures. For a radiologist of the old school, interventional radiology was the most startling innovation of all, for it meant changing from being "a doctor's doctor" to a caregiver. In the 1980s interventional radiology meant moving from conventional angiography, involving injecting radio-opaque substances directly into blood vessels, to therapeutic procedures in the vascular tree and elsewhere. Toronto had several pioneers of these techniques.

The true pioneer of interventional angiography in Toronto was Ron Colapinto at the Toronto General Hospital. In 1977 Colapinto began making liver biopsies safer by pushing a catheter down the jugular vein to the hepatic vein and thus into the liver.[44] This technique had been previously described, but Colapinto improved it by inventing a new needle (the "Colapinto needle") that reduced the friction of the needle against the catheter wall by simply placing the bevel of the needle on the other side.[45]

Next he tried using the catheter to embolize bleeding varices, which otherwise were approachable only surgically through the abdomen. One evening around 1980 as he sat explaining the biopsy technique "to a couple of residents," the idea of an internal shunt struck him. If the biopsy needle went the wrong direction into the main hepatic vein (risking bursting through into the portal vein), it might be good rather than bad. "The beauty of it was," he later said, "that the patient couldn't bleed to death because the hole you were making was between the portal vein and the hepatic vein. From one vein to the other, so any bleeding that occurred was still in the vascular system."

Then he exclaimed to himself, "In fact if it happened it would help decompress the portal system and be like a shunt!" He sat there thinking. "If we could make that hole bigger we would have a shunt."

At the time they had started to do angioplasty of the legs using a balloon catheter. Colapinto said, "Why don't we try putting a balloon down and enlarging the hole purposely and see if blood will flow from the portal vein?" He spoke with the surgeons and they agreed.

So in 1981 they began ramming the balloon catheter "right through the liver from one vein into the other vein, so that the blood will flow from the portal system to the vena cava." Until then they had been doing this with a 3 mm. needle. With an 8 or 10 mm. balloon "we could make a big hole between those two veins. That's basically what the surgery is when they go in and do surgically a shunt. The trouble is, if it's done in an emergency situation the mortality rate is about 75 percent. So it wasn't a great surgical procedure." But Colapinto's TIPS, or Transjugular Intrahepatic Portosystemic Shunt, reduced the mortality to 25 percent. Of the twenty patients on whom they attempted TIPS between 1981 and 1985, 15 survived (another three lived more than six months).

The next logical step was to insert a metal tube, or stent, through the liver in order to keep the hole open. This was almost a Toronto story. The San Antonio radiologist Julio Palmaz had fashioned an appropriate stent. He phoned Colapinto and said, "Would you like to be the first one to put one of these stents in, since you did the first TIPS procedure?"

"Sure," said Colapinto.

"Next time you have one, I'll fly up with a stent and we'll put it in," said Palmaz.

The trouble was that, as Colapinto put it, "all the patients we were doing were acute emergencies at four in the morning. I was never able to say, 'We're going to do one tomorrow afternoon. Come on up.' So we just missed putting in the first stent."

Colapinto had not just limited himself to the abdomen. Until the mid-1970s he had done occasional cerebral procedures as well. When neuroradiologist Richard Holgate arrived in Toronto in the mid-1970s, he was cross-appointed at the General and began doing neurointerventional procedures there. Said Colapinto with mock surliness, "Yeah, he took the business away from me." Colapinto and Holgate therefore mark the beginning of neurointerventional radiology in Toronto.

When in 1984 Holgate resigned to take a post in South Carolina, Gordon Potts had just been appointed, and the crisis at the Toronto Western Hospital was just unfolding. Potts opened a new chapter in the history of neurointerventional radiology in Toronto when he identified for leadership a staff radiologist at Toronto Western Hospital named Karel TerBrugge. TerBrugge was born in 1945 in Holland, became MD at the University of Utrecht in 1968 and, after a rotating internship at Utrecht, came to the Toronto Western Hospital in 1970 to do another rotating internship and get a Canadian license. TerBrugge trained in diagnostic radiology at the Western until 1975, then fellowed in neuroradiology at the Montreal Neurological Institute. From 1988 on, TerBrugge was head of neuroradiology at the Western. It was Potts's plan that the gifted young TerBrugge make TWH a prominent center in neuroradiology. "I implemented his idea," said TerBrugge modestly later. "Potts was a very forward-looking, a very wise person who could see into the future. He had ideas truly at the professorial level." Potts's idea was that TerBrugge would help "build a complement of young people in neuroradiology at the Western who felt comfortable in this environment," as TerBrugge put it.

It was, however, TerBrugge himself who, along with his colleague Ming-Chai Chiu, had targeted interventional procedures as the side of neuroradiology the Western was to move forward in. "We got [neurosurgeon] Alan Hudson to endorse a one-center-in-Toronto approach. So from the outset we had the neurosurgeons with us."[46]

The story goes back to the early 1980s when Harnick was still chief and Chiu the head of neuroradiology. Chiu and TerBrugge agreed that they wanted to begin a neurointerventional program at the Western, but did not know quite how to go about it. Chiu said later, "I was doing embolization on a trial basis by reading journals and going to meetings, but I was never properly taught." Chiu and TerBrugge agreed they should bring somebody in to teach them, and in 1983 identified the Parisian neuroradiologist Pierre Lasjaunias, a world leader in the embolization of cerebral vascular lesions, as the person. Although Harnick himself never saw much of a role for radiology beyond providing service to other departments, he agreed on the Western's need for Lasjaunias. Harnick intervened with the hospital to fund the move, with the College to grant an educational license, and with the university to offer Lasjaunias an academic post.[47]

In 1984 Chiu and TerBrugge created a formal program in interventional neuroradiological techniques at the Western. Lasjaunias spent a six-month sabbatical in Toronto, then began flying back and forth on a quarterly basis. With Chiu and TerBrugge assisting, Lasjaunias would perform "sophisticated endovascular treatment procedures for brain and spinal cord arteriovenous malformations," as TerBrugge later described it.[48] When Potts became chief of the hospital department in 1985, it was well positioned to make a major effort in the neurointerventional field. After 1988 TerBrugge himself, now the head of neuroradiology at the Western, had become skilled enough to work as a "supervising person" with other fledgling interventional neuroradiology programs in Canada, such as the Montreal Neurological Institute at McGill. TerBrugge began taking on fellows in diagnostic and therapeutic neuroradiology from other centers and between 1988 and 1994 trained twelve of them at the Western. By 1993 TerBrugge and the Interventional Neuroradiology Program at The Toronto Hospital were receiving referrals from all over Canada, and represented the foremost Canadian center for this subspecialty.

Walter Kucharczyk noted the irony of changing the name of the department to "medical imaging" in 1994. Once again, radiology was becoming a therapeutic discipline. "For example, balloon angioplasty of stenotic vessels, placement of portal-systemic stents, percutaneous abscess drainage, percutaneous stone removal, endovascular obliteration of cerebroaneurysms and vascular malformations: all are procedures we perform. Indeed, just as we wound down our responsibilities in therapeutic radiation over the past three decades, we markedly increased the number of minimally invasive procedures we perform today based on accurate image guidance."[49] In a hundred years of radiology, the wheel was coming a full circle.

What began in 1896 in Toronto as the study of "Roentgen Rays" had ended a century later as a very different discipline. Yet the term radiology has a comfortable feel. When in 1982 the radiology department at St. Michael's Hospital was contemplating changing its name to "medical imaging," chief radiologist Bruce Bird said that he felt the change was appropriate enough, and that he had no objections provided the hospital signs could still state "X-ray" for the benefit of the public. But Dr. Bird said tongue-in-cheek that he was "not too enthusiastic about the title Medical Imager-in-Chief."[50]

Indeed the men and women who have transformed this specialty from looking at the play of shadows from a Crookes tube to embolizing arteriovenous malformations with injections of a glue-like substance still refer to themselves as "radiologists." But the story of radiology in Toronto has taken them from kindly old Dr. Edmund King, examining the lesions of the poor street-corner fluoroscoper, to a sprawling university department involving eight hospitals, over a hundred faculty, and almost as many residents and fellows.[51] These are solid achievements. From the progress of science can flow great benefits.

Endnotes

[1] TGH MAB, Feb. 26, 1948. Dauphinee was cross-appointed to the university's Department of Pathological Chemistry.

[2] See TWH MAB, Nov. 15, 1949. The Toronto Western Hospital sent Dr. Brown as its liaison person. See also W. G. Cosbie, *The Toronto General Hospital, 1819-1965: A Chronicle* (Toronto: Macmillan, 1975), pp. 252-253. Also: James A. Dauphinee, "The Clinical Use of Isotopes," OCTRF, *Annual Report 1949,* pp. 73-74.

[3] K. J. R. Wightman, "Report to the Medical Advisory Board Re: Isotope Facilities in the New Hospital," attached to TGH MAB, May 21, 1953. Ash belonged to the committee that produced this report, yet Ash may have been thinking about the future Ontario Cancer Institute and not about the turf struggles of the Department of Radiology at TGH.

[4] TGH MAB, Feb. 17, 1955.

[5] For a concise account, see Ronald L. Eisenberg, *Radiology: An Illustrated History* (St. Louis: Mosby, 1992), see pp. 417-419.

[6] Bernard Shapiro interview of Jan. 24, 1995.

[7] Department of Radiology, "Presentation to Interdepartmental Planning Co-ordination Committee, Toronto General Hospital," May 25, 1966, pp. 29-30.

[8] TGH Trustees, Jan. 17, 1968, p. 2780; TGH MAB, May 20, 1971.

[9] *Report of the Dean, 1970-71,* p. 156. The TGH staff list for 1970-71 reflects these arrangements.

[10] HSC MAB, Jan. 11, 1956.

[11] HSC MAB, Apr. 6, 1966, re "Recommendations by Dr. C. A. F. Moes for proposed establishment of a radioactive isotope committee."

[12] HSC MAB, Feb. 5, 1969.

[13] HSC MAB, Dec. 1, 1971.

[14] HSC MAB, Mar. 1, 1972; see changes to the staff list for 1972.

[15] [HSC] *What's New,* Feb. 1975, p. 4.

[16] MSH Executive Committee, Nov. 3, 1967.

[17] See H. Patrick Higgins and William Singer, "The History of the Department of Nuclear Medicine at St. Michael's Hospital," 1981; manuscript in SMH Archives.

[18] Shapiro interview. "What's all this s—— about nukes and ultrasound?" Harnick said to Shapiro once. "X-rays is what we ought to do."

[19] See Lansdown to Gilday, Aug. 3, 1979; Lansdown to Holmes, Dec. 4, 1979; in Lansdown Papers.

[20] See TGH Trustees, May 12 and June 9, 1981; Feb. 9, 1982.

[21] Potts interview, Feb. 2, 1994.

[22] Interview with Sylvain Houle of Feb. 21, 1995.

[23] RCPS, "Report of the Specialty Committee in Diagnostic Radiology," May 23, 1975, p. 4.

[24] "Ad Hoc Committee on Ultra Sound," Aug. 15, 1977. SMH Archives.

[25] George Wortzman interview of Dec. 14, 1994.

[26] "Department of Radiology, Faculty of Medicine, University of Toronto, Departmental Survey," 1979, entry under TWH, p. 3. In Lansdown Papers.

[27] On Hounsfield, EMI, and the development of CT scanning, see Stuart S. Blume, *Insight and Industry: On the Dynamics of Technological Change in Medicine* (Cambridge: MIT, 1992), pp. 159-172.

[28]"Proceedings of the British Institute of Radiology: Abstracts of Papers Read at the 32nd Annual Congress, April 20-21, 1972," *British Journal of Radiology*, 46 (Feb. 1973), pp. 147-149.

[29]Gordon Potts, personal communication.

[30]Much of the following is based on an interview with Holmes, April 20, 1995.

[31]See the listing of the "Symposium: New Technologies in Radiology," in the program of the RSNA, published in *Radiology*, 105 (1972), p. 215.

[32]See TGH Trustees, July 11, Aug. 8, Oct. 10, 1973; Feb. 6, 1974.

[33]TGH MAB, Oct. 7, 1976, appendix A.

[34]For some details see Sister Camilla to C. G. Gonsalves, Jan. 29, 1976; SMH Archives.

[35]SMH MAB, Jan. 10, 1977.

[36]See SMH MAB, Mar. 6, 1978, "Equipment Purchase Committee Allocation for Fiscal 1978/79." $370,000 had been budgeted for "scanner up-date." The equipment budget was $350,000.

[37]Department of Radiology, *Annual Report, 1992-1993*, passim.

[38]TGH Trustees, Nov. 8, 1983, pp. 5921-22.

[39]TGH Trustees, May 9, 1984, pp. 6066-67.

[40]TGH Trustees, Sept. 11, 1984, p. 6132.

[41]TGH MAB, Mar. 17, 1983.

[42]TGH MAB, Apr. 7, 1983.

[43]"Super Magnet Looks Through Body," *Toronto Star*, Feb. 11, 1987, p. A3.

[44]Ronald Colapinto interview of Mar. 2, 1995. See his "Transjugular Biopsy of the Liver," *Clinics in Gastroenterology*, 14 (2) (Apr. 1985), pp. 451-467.

[45]Ronald F. Colapinto and L. M. Blendis, "A Modified Needle for Transjugular Biopsy of the Liver," *Radiology*, 148 (1983), p. 306. I rely for my chronology of these events on some lectures notes Colapinto kindly shared with me, entitled "TIPS: Early Canadian Experience."

[46]Interview with Karel TerBrugge of Mar. 21, 1995.

[47]Interview with Ming-Chai Chiu of May 9, 1995.

[48]Department of Radiology, *Annual Report, 1987-1988*, p. 65.

[49]Walter Kucharczyk, personal communication.

[50]SMC MAB, Aug. 30, 1982.

[51]Department of Radiology, *Annual Report, 1990-1991*, p. 1.

Index

A

Abbe, Robert, 34
academic radiology, 7, 65, 140-141
  and Royal College fellowship, 124-125
  vs. community service, 94
Acta-Scanner (CT scanner), 159
Aikens, W. H. B. ("Henry"), 33-34
air encephalography, 72, 85
Albert Einstein College of Medicine, New
  York, 156
Allison, Ruth, *photo*, p. 103
Allt, William, 46
Ambrose, James, 157
American Board of Nuclear Medicine
  diploma, 150
American College of Radiology, 67
American Radium Society, 34
American Society for Therapeutic Radiology
  and Oncology, 47, 56
American Society of Neuroradiology, 73, 86,
  113
Anderson, Harry B., 88
Anger, Hal, 148
angiography, 73-76, 82, 98, 134-135, 162
  coronary, 91
  diagnostic x-ray camera, 82
angioplasty, 163
anti-Semitism, 105
  in residency appointments, 129
Archives of Ontario, xi
Armed Forces Institute, Washington, 74
Armed Forces Radiology Course, 69
Art Gallery of Toronto, 89
arteriography, 72
Arts and Letters Club, 24, 89
Ash, Clifford, 42-49, 53, 57, 59, 65, 131, 147
  biography and character, 42-43, *photo*, p. 43
Ash, Judith, 44
Association of Canadian Medical Colleges, 137
Association of University Radiologists, 67
Atkinson Foundation, 97
Atkinson Morley's Hospital, 142

B

B____, Hattie R., 14
Banting Institute, radioactive isotope
  laboratory, 148

Banting, Sir Frederick, 103-104
Banting, Henrietta, 103, *photo*, p. 103
Barker, Lewellys, 127
Battle Creek Sanatarium, Michigan, 92
Bell-Milburn, Helen
  See Milburn, Helen (Bell-)
Bellevue Hospital, New York, 100
Beschai, Nabil, 96
betatron, 57-58
Beth Tzedec Congregation, 93
Bigelow, W. G. ("Bill"), 77
biomedical engineering, 152
biplane angiographic unit, 95
Bird, Bruce, 91, 97-98, 129, 138, 166
Bird, Grant, 91, 97-98
Blackwell, Frederick N., 126
Blackwell, C. S., 19
Blair, Allan, 41, 58
"blue babies", 82
Bonner, Keith, 97
Boston Children's Hospital, 7
Boston City Hospital, 84
Branscombe family, 159
breast cancer, 37, 39-40, 44, 50, 53, 102
  lumpectomy, 53-54
  radiation therapy, 53-54
  radical mastectomy, 53
Briggs, G. A., 5
British Columbia Cancer Institute, 102
British Empire Cancer Campaign
  Fellowship, 43
British Medical Journal, 12
Brown, Alan, 25, 128
Brown, Donald, 111
Brown, John, 57
Bruce, Herbert A., 38, 96
Burhenne, Joachim, 141
Burke, Desmond, 110-111
Burrow, Gerald, 154

C

Caffey, John, 81
Calgary General Hospital, 25
Cambridge University, 123
Campbell, John, 113-114
Canadian army hospital, Basingstoke,
  England, 23
Canadian Association of Nuclear Medicine, 151

Index

174